WARD LOCK

FAMILY HEALTH GUID

FIRST AID

CW00747625

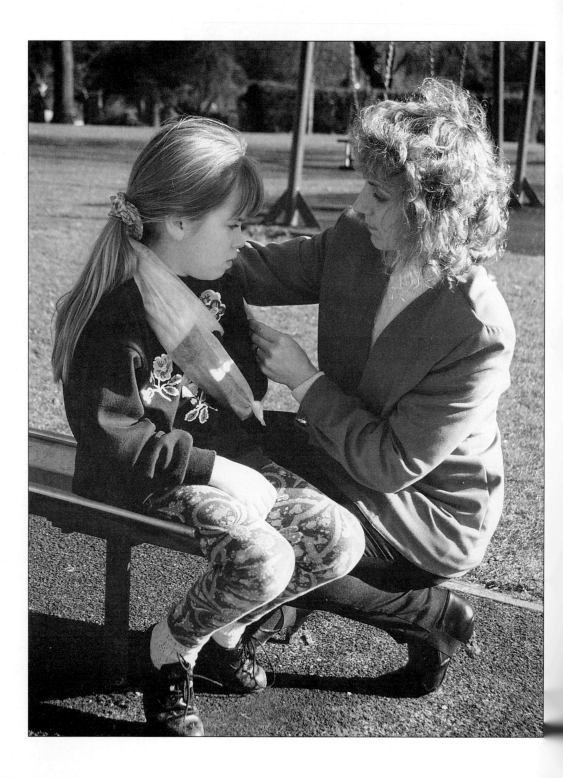

WARD LOCK

FAMILY HEALTH GUIDE

FIRST AID

DR ANDREW MASON

PRODUCED WITH THE HELP OF THE
BRITISH ASSOCIATION FOR IMMEDIATE CARE

WARD LOCK

Dr Andrew M. Mason
Dr Andrew Mason MB, BS, MRCS,LRCP is a Lecturer and Examiner in First Aid for the British Red Cross Society and St John Ambulance Brigade. He is also an Examiner in First Aid for Eastern Electricity plc, and a Lecturer in Cardiology on the Paramedic Training Scheme of the East Anglian Ambulance NHS Trust.

Design and content of this book
This book covers all common medical emergencies that may be encountered in the home, at school or in the workplace. Technical terms have been kept to a minimum and no previous First Aid experience has been assumed. All the resuscitation techniques comply with the 1992 standards set by the Working Party of the European Resuscitation Council, and the book should prove to be an invaluable source of reference for any home.

A WARD LOCK BOOK

First published in the UK 1994
by Ward Lock
Villiers House
41/47 Strand
London
WC2N 5JE

A Cassell Imprint

Designed and produced
by SP Creative Design
147 Kings Road, Bury St Edmunds, Suffolk, England
Editor: Heather Thomas
Art director: Rolando Ugolini
Illustrations: Rolando Ugolini

Distributed in the United States
by Sterling Publishing Co., Inc.
387 Park Avenue South, New York, NY 10016-8810

Distributed in Australia
by Capricorn Link(Australia) Pty Ltd
2/13 Carrington Road, Castle Hill, NSW 2154

A British Library Cataloguing in Publication Data block for this book may be obtained from the British Library.

ISBN 0 7063 7254 9

Printed and bound in Spain

Acknowledgements
The author wishes to acknowledge the assistance given by Dr Judith M. Fisher, MB BS FRCGP, Keith Hotchkiss, SEN, and members of the Bury St Edmunds divisions of the British Red Cross Society and St John Ambulance Brigade in preparing this book.

Contents

Introduction

"Saving life is a matter for the layman, less important matters we can leave to doctors."
(Kurt Hahn: 1886-1974)

Definition

First Aid is the initial assistance or treatment given to an injured or sick person before professional medical care becomes available.

The purpose of First Aid

Purpose	Example
1 To preserve life	Giving mouth-to-mouth ventilation when breathing has stopped
2 To prevent a worsening of the problem	Stopping an untrained bystander from moving a casualty when it is not necessary
3 To promote healing and recovery	Cleaning and disinfecting a dirty wound

Practice makes perfect

Skills, such as applying an arm sling, can be practised at home with the help of a friend prepared to act as a casualty. However, certain procedures, such as 'heart massage' (external chest compression), cannot be performed on volunteers since to do so could be dangerous. In order to get around this problem, a variety of life-sized dummies (manikins) have been specially created. Resuscitation manikins are used on all public First Aid courses in the UK run by voluntary organisations such as the British Red Cross Society and St John Ambulance Brigade (St Andrew's Ambulance Association in Scotland), and it must be stressed that there is no satisfactory substitute for this type of 'hands on' experience.

Equipment

When dealing with an injury, access to a First Aid kit can be a great help (see page 78), but a good First Aider should be able to substitute items that come readily to hand, e.g. a clean handkerchief to control bleeding from a wound, or a scarf to act as a temporary sling. In any case, the basic resuscitation techniques detailed in this book require no special equipment and, once learnt, can be employed in a wide range of emergency situations.

Part one

Dealing with an emergency

 ## Safety first

Before attempting to give emergency assistance to an injured person, it is essential that you take account of any local hazards such as electricity, fire and moving traffic. If an unwary First Aider simply becomes another casualty, the situation is made worse, so personal safety must always take priority.

When dealing with an emergency, you should try to remain calm. This not only helps you to think more clearly, but also enables you to gain the confidence of your patient and any bystanders. Every accident is unique and it requires a lot of practice to become a good First Aider. Nevertheless, some basic First Aid knowledge coupled with common sense will often be enough to secure a satisfactory outcome.

However, you should:

- Always be aware of your limitations.
- Never attempt too much.
- Be prepared to make way for someone who is more experienced.

Making a diagnosis

A diagnosis is simply a judgement of what is wrong with a patient. In an emergency, it is sometimes difficult to make an accurate diagnosis and even doctors may need the help of special tests (e.g. an X-ray to confirm that a bone is broken). Although it is useful to know the precise nature of the problem, it is far more important that the First Aider should be able to recognise life-threatening conditions, such as a blocked airway, failure to breathe, cardiac arrest and severe bleeding, and to take prompt and appropriate action. Making a diagnosis can be aided by:

- Taking a history.
- Asking about symptoms.
- Identifying signs.
- Finding external clues.

History

A medical history is an account of the circumstances leading up to, and surrounding, the incident – how the accident happened or the illness began – and may be obtained directly from the patient, or from a bystander. Try to find out the casualty's name, age and address. Ask about previous medical problems and find out if any medication is being taken. Write any important facts down.

7

Dealing with an emergency

Symptoms

Symptoms are feelings experienced by the patient, e.g. pain, dizziness, nausea, numbness etc. These will not be obtainable if the patient is unconscious.

Signs

Signs are things that you can detect using any of your own senses. For example, you can see a bruise, smell alcohol on the breath, hear wheezing or feel a swelling.

External clues

These include items carried or worn by the patient alerting you to the existence of medical problems such as diabetes, epilepsy and allergies. If the casualty is unconscious or uncooperative, search through pockets or belongings and keep a look out for lockets, pendants or bracelets with the markings 'Medic-Alert' or 'SOS Talisman'; these may provide vital information. The finding of a syringe could mean that the patient is a diabetic or a drug abuser, and tablets or a hospital appointment card can sometimes indicate what may be wrong. Draw your findings to the attention of ambulance personnel or doctors, and do not allow any items to become separated from the patient.

Making a 999 call in the UK

The 999 system is a free service, so no money or phonecard is needed when making emergency calls from a public telephone. The operator will ask you which emergency service you require (Police, Fire, Ambulance or Coastguard) and the number you are calling from. Sometimes two or more of these services are needed at an incident, e.g. the Police, a Fire Service rescue vehicle and an ambulance will be needed if an injured person is trapped in a vehicle following a road accident. If anyone is injured or seriously ill, you should always ask to be put through to the Ambulance Service.

The Ambulance Control Officer who talks to you, will request the following information:

- The location of the emergency.
- The nature of the incident.
- The number of casualties.
- Whether any people are trapped.
- Whether there are any hazards such as fire (other emergency services will be alerted automatically if they are needed).
- Your name, address and telephone number.
- Any additional information (e.g. the name of the casualty, if known).
- Do not replace the receiver until the Controller has cleared the line.

If you send someone else to telephone for help, first ask them to repeat the message so that you can check that it is complete and accurate, and instruct them to return immediately afterwards to report that the call has been received.

Clear a space around the casualty for the ambulance crew and, if necessary, ensure that someone waits at the roadside to signal the location where help is required.

Helping accident victims

	Action	Notes
V	View the scene and verify that it is safe to approach.	Ask witnesses what happened. Be aware of hazards such as live cables, fire, gas, unstable structures and moving traffic. Keep yourself and others back if the risks appear too great. Remove any dangers from around the victim and only move the casualty as a last resort.
I	Inspect the injuries.	Make a quick assessment of the number of casualties and the injuries involved. Examine the most seriously injured first (often these will be the quiet ones). If anyone is unconscious, follow the **ABC** of resuscitation (see pages 10-31).
C	Call for help.	If help is needed, shout for assistance or telephone.
T	Treat the condition.	**ABC** of resuscitation takes priority. Then deal with severe bleeding. Next stabilize any broken bones if the casualty needs to be moved. If a spinal injury is suspected, only move if other dangers threaten life. Finally treat any minor injuries.
I	Inform the patient.	Communicate with your patient throughout and reassure regularly. Always explain what you are about to do. It is good practice to talk to casualties even if you suspect they may be unconscious.
M	Monitor the patient's condition.	Keep a careful watch on all vital signs. Regularly check the breathing and pulse and be prepared to follow the **ABC** of resuscitation if necessary.
S	Stay with your patient.	Do not leave your patient before help arrives. Be ready to pass on any relevant information. If you have had time to make notes, hand these over.

Dealing with an emergency

ABC of resuscitation

Our bodies need a regular supply of oxygen. This is present in the air we breathe and finds its way into the bloodstream through the network of tiny blood vessels surrounding the air sacs (alveoli) in the lungs.

As oxygen passes from the air sacs into the bloodstream, carbon dioxide travels in

Oxygen enters the bloodstream in the lungs

Artery

Vein

Bronchiole

Alveolus (air sac)

Network of capillaries cover alveoli

the opposite direction, and this waste product is flushed out every time we breath out. The oxygenated blood collects in the pulmonary veins and the beating heart then distributes it around the body. If deprived of oxygen, all living tissues will eventually die, but the brain is particularly sensitive to

ABC – the priorities of first aid

In order to keep the brain supplied with oxygen, there must be:

 a clear Airway to allow oxygen-containing air to reach the lungs

 adequate Breathing to allow the blood in the lungs to be replenished with oxygen

 an effective Circulation of blood to distribute oxygen around the body.

oxygen-lack and begins to suffer permanent damage within three or four minutes of the supply being interrupted. In less than ten minutes the brain may be totally destroyed with no prospect of any recovery.

Resuscitation

Resuscitation is the term used for the emergency action required when there is a failure of one or more of the above functions. This may involve clearing an obstruction from the airway of someone who is choking, giving the mouth to mouth ventilation ('kiss-of-life') to someone who has stopped breathing, or applying external chest compression ('heart massage') when the heart stops beating. These resuscitation techniques (referred to collectively as cardio-pulmonary resuscitation, or CPR) can be performed without the need for any special equipment, and saving a life can be as easy as knowing your **ABC**. Remember that, if resuscitation is needed, it is important to act quickly – seconds really do count when the brain is starved of oxygen.

Safety first

Always remember to check that it is safe to approach the casualty. Be aware of the dangers from electricity, gas, fire and fumes, falling masonry and other unstable objects, moving traffic etc. **Remember that personal safety must always take priority.**

Assess the level of consciousness

Eliminate any continuing danger (e.g. by switching off an electrical supply) and then determine the casualty's state of consciousness. This can be done by grasping the shoulders and shaking them gently, whilst calling out, 'Are you all right?'

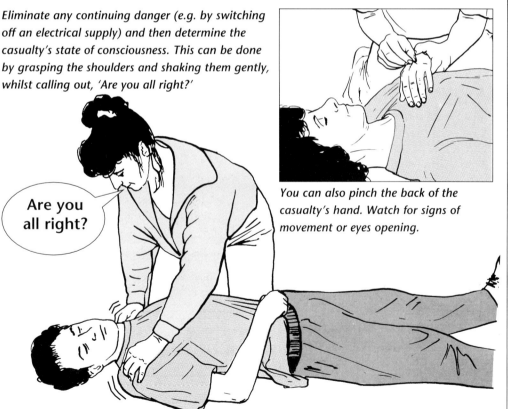

Are you all right?

You can also pinch the back of the casualty's hand. Watch for signs of movement or eyes opening.

Dealing with an emergency

If the casualty is conscious, start by controlling any severe bleeding (see page 37), then support or stabilize any fractures (see page 61). Do not move the casualty unless he is in immediate danger. If help is needed, shout for assistance or telephone, and then treat any minor injuries. Monitor the breathing and pulse and be prepared to follow the **ABC** of resuscitation. Semi-conscious patients may groan or move slightly, or you may notice a flickering of the eyelids. They should be treated as if they were unconscious.

Airway

In the unconscious state, the muscles sag in the mouth and throat and this can lead to a narrowing of the airway. The situation is aggravated if the unconscious casualty is lying on his back since, in this position, gravity causes the tongue to fall against the back of the throat and this may completely obstruct the airway. Other things that may block the airway include water or weeds in cases of near-drowning, chunks of food when someone is choking, or blood, vomit, broken dentures etc. Because the tongue is attached to the jawbone, lifting the chin will help to pull the tongue clear of the back of the throat. The airway can be further widened by gently extending the neck, but extreme care should be exercised if neck injuries are suspected (see pages 71-73). Opening the airway in this manner is often all that is needed to allow normal breathing to resume.

If the airway remains blocked, quickly inspect inside the mouth. In adults, finger sweeps can be tried in an attempt to hook out solid obstructions such as broken

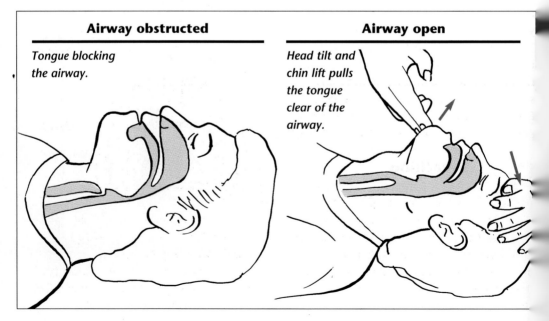

Airway obstructed

Tongue blocking the airway.

Airway open

Head tilt and chin lift pulls the tongue clear of the airway.

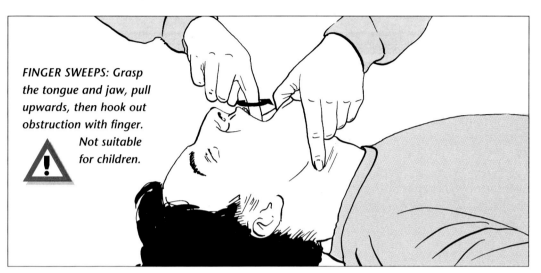

FINGER SWEEPS: Grasp the tongue and jaw, pull upwards, then hook out obstruction with finger. Not suitable for children.

dentures or chunks of food, but care should be taken to avoid pushing anything further down the throat. Liquids like blood and vomit can be scooped out with the aid of a handkerchief wrapped around the index and middle fingers, but don't twist the neck if you think there may be neck injuries.

If breathing returns but the casualty remains unconscious, do a head-to-toe check for life-threatening injuries, remove any sharp items of jewellery, spectacles, keys from pockets etc., turn him into the recovery position (see pages 25-26) and send for help.

Breathing

Each time we inhale, muscles attached to our ribs act to expand the chest. At the same time a sheet of muscle called the diaphragm pulls downwards. Providing there is no blockage in the airway, air gets sucked into the lungs and is then expelled simply by the elastic recoil of the ribcage as the breathing

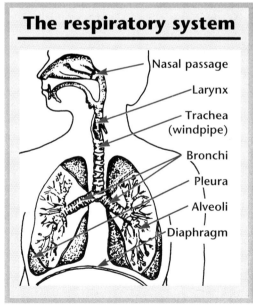

The respiratory system

Nasal passage
Larynx
Trachea (windpipe)
Bronchi
Pleura
Alveoli
Diaphragm

muscles relax. Normally we take a breath around 16 times-a-minute.

To check if an unconscious casualty is breathing, we need to **look**, **listen** and **feel**. Whilst kneeling beside the casualty, facing his

13

Dealing with an emergency

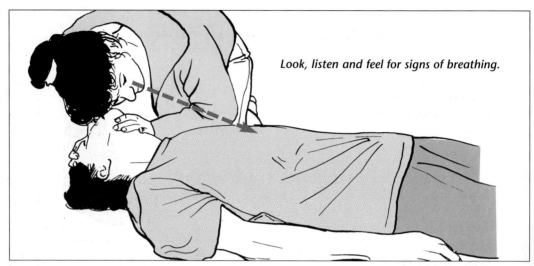

Look, listen and feel for signs of breathing.

feet, place your ear close to his mouth and:
- **Look** for a rise and fall of the chest or abdomen.
- **Listen** for breath sounds.
- **Feel** for breath on your face (this is helped by moistening your cheek).

In cold weather you may even notice vapour escaping from the casualty's mouth.

If breathing is adequate, perform a body check, treat any life-threatening condition, and prepare to place him in the recovery position (see pages 25-26). If breathing cannot be detected, you should immediately check the circulation by feeling for the carotid pulse in the neck.

Circulation

Every time the heart beats (normally around 60 or 70 times a minute at rest), it sends a quantity of blood into the main artery of the body – the aorta. Valves in the heart prevent blood leaking back between beats, so the blood is continually nudged down the aorta and into the smaller arteries which branch off it. The pressure wave produced each time the heart contracts makes the walls of the arteries expand briefly, accounting for the pulse that can be felt over an artery.

When a casualty is in shock, the pulse will be weak and may easily be missed if taken at the wrist. For this reason, it is the carotid pulse that should be checked in adults to find out if the heart is beating. To locate the carotid pulse, gently place your index and middle fingers on top of the casualty's voice box, and then slide them down into the groove between the voice box and the muscles that run along the side of the neck. With the pads of the fingers (not the tips as these are less sensitive), feel here for around 5 seconds.

If the casualty is unconscious and has no pulse, the heart has stopped (cardiac arrest) and immediate action will be needed to support both breathing and circulation.

14

Finding the carotid pulse

The carotid artery lies in the groove between the windpipe and muscles of the neck.

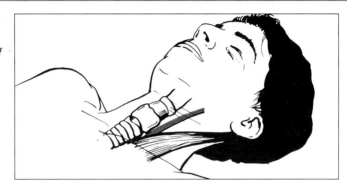

1 Whilst keeping the head tilted, place the tips of your fingers over the casualty's voice box (larynx).

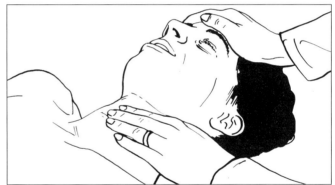

2 Slide the tips of your fingers down the side of the larynx into the groove of the neck between the windpipe and neck muscles and apply gentle pressure to feel for the pulse in the artery.

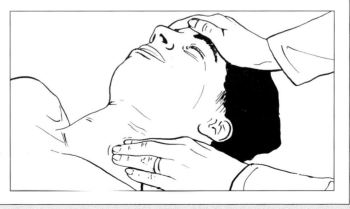

Dealing with an emergency

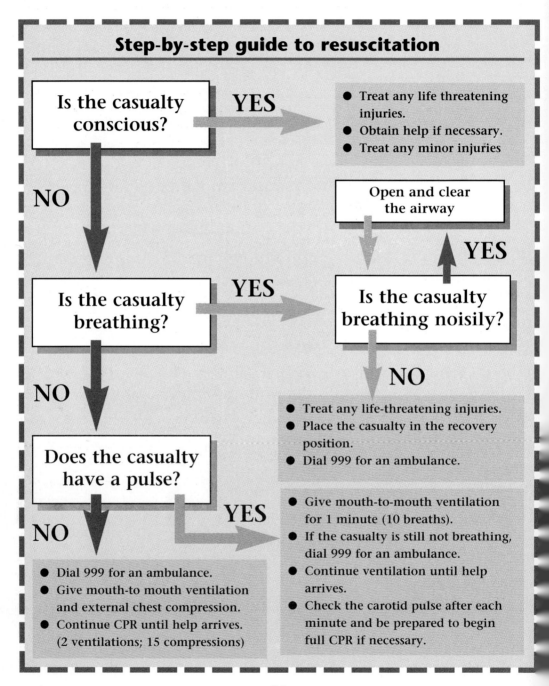

Step-by-step guide to resuscitation

Is the casualty conscious?

YES
- Treat any life threatening injuries.
- Obtain help if necessary.
- Treat any minor injuries

NO

Open and clear the airway

Is the casualty breathing?

YES → **Is the casualty breathing noisily?**

YES ↑

NO
- Treat any life-threatening injuries.
- Place the casualty in the recovery position.
- Dial 999 for an ambulance.

NO

Does the casualty have a pulse?

YES
- Give mouth-to-mouth ventilation for 1 minute (10 breaths).
- If the casualty is still not breathing, dial 999 for an ambulance.
- Continue ventilation until help arrives.
- Check the carotid pulse after each minute and be prepared to begin full CPR if necessary.

NO
- Dial 999 for an ambulance.
- Give mouth-to mouth ventilation and external chest compression.
- Continue CPR until help arrives. (2 ventilations; 15 compressions)

Mouth-to-mouth ventilation ('kiss of life')

Although our bodies use up oxygen, there is still enough oxygen in the air we breathe out to keep someone else alive.

In order to perform mouth-to-mouth ventilation, the casualty should be lying on his back and you should be kneeling alongside his head. However, you should not be deterred from attempting the procedure if a casualty is trapped in another position. The instructions that follow apply to adults in whom a pulse is present. For the resuscitation of children, see pages 27-31.

EMERGENCY ACTION

1 First loosen any tight clothing, then open the airway by tilting the head back and lifting the chin. Quickly inspect inside the mouth and clear any obvious obstruction, but leave well-fitting dentures in place; these help to create a good mouth-to-mouth seal. With the airway held open, look, listen and feel for signs of breathing.

2 In the absence of breathing but with a pulse present, pinch the casualty's nostrils between the thumb and index finger of one hand, whilst controlling the chin with your other hand. Now take a deep breath and prepare to seal your lips firmly around the open mouth.

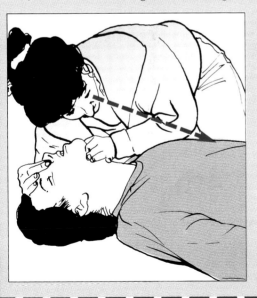
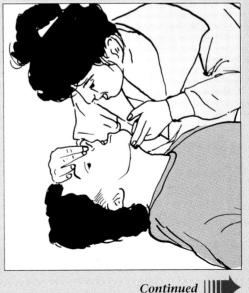

Continued ||||▶

17

Dealing with an emergency

◀▐▐▐ *Continued from page 17*

3 Breathe firmly into the mouth and, at the same time, look along the line of the chest to check that it rises. Try to blow smoothly over a period of a couple of seconds until you see the chest rise.

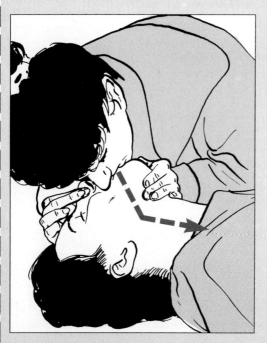

4 Take your mouth away but maintain the head tilt/chin lift position with your hands. Watch for the chest to fall by elastic recoil, which should take between 2 and 4 seconds.

5 If you feel resistance when you blow and you are having difficulty in getting the chest to rise, first try tilting the head further back as the commonest cause of obstruction is an inadequately-opened airway. If the chest still fails to rise, assume that there is a foreign body blocking the airway and perform finger sweeps (N.B. **not** suitable for children). Do this by grasping both the tongue and lower jaw between your thumb and index finger and pulling upwards. This draws the tongue from the back of the throat and may reveal a foreign body previously overlooked. With one or two fingers of the other hand sweep around behind the object and hook it out, taking care not to push it further down the throat.

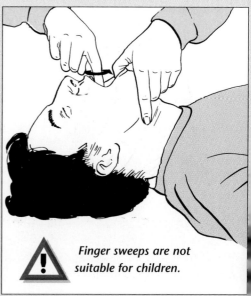

⚠ *Finger sweeps are not suitable for children.*

6 If you fail to relieve the obstruction with finger sweeps, turn the casualty onto his side by rolling him towards you, and deliver up to five firm slaps between the shoulder blades, followed by finger sweeps. If the airway remains obstructed you must immediately perform abdominal thrusts (Heimlich manoeuvre). With the casualty lying on his back, kneel astride his hips and place the heel of one hand slightly above the tummy button with the fingertips just below the ribcage. Put your other hand on top and deliver one or more quick upward thrusts. The aim is to force the diaphragm upwards to expel the obstruction like a cork from a popgun. Several thrusts may be necessary to dislodge a foreign body, which may then be hooked out of the mouth using a finger sweep.

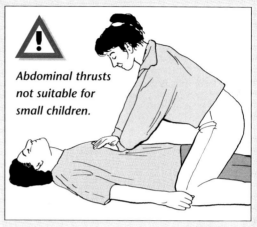

Abdominal thrusts not suitable for small children.

BLOCKED AIRWAY - If finger sweeps and back slaps are unsuccessful, use abdominal thrusts (Heimlich manoeuvre)

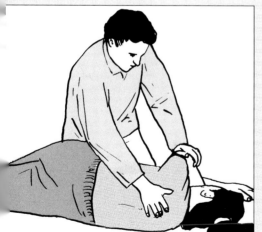

If finger sweeps do not relieve the obstruction, give up to five back slaps.

7 When the obstruction is relieved, check the carotid pulse and, providing the heart is still beating, give ten mouth-to-mouth ventilations over the course of the next minute (one breath every six seconds). If breathing has not returned within the first minute, send someone to telephone 999 for an ambulance. If you have to make the call yourself, make every effort to be back within two or three minutes. If the casualty is still not breathing, continue ventilating at a rate of one breath every six seconds until breathing returns. Check the pulse at the end of each minute and be prepared to start external chest compressions if the pulse disappears. When normal breathing and colour return, place the casualty in the recovery position (see pages 25-26).

Dealing with an emergency

Circulation

Cardiac arrest

If the heart stops beating, oxygenated blood no longer reaches the vital organs and there is a risk of permanent brain damage in as little as three or four minutes. Sudden cardiac arrest may occur in the early stages of a 'heart attack' (myocardial infarct) or following an electric shock, and the casualty loses consciousness almost immediately. The pulse disappears and breathing ceases soon afterwards, although an occasional gasp may be noticed for up to about minute. During this time there may well be some twitching of the body, and the lips, earlobes and nailbeds may start to turn blue. Lack of oxygen to the brain causes the pupils to enlarge although, if brain damage is not too severe, they will still constrict in response to bright light.

Following a cardiac arrest, immediate action is needed if brain damage is to be prevented. Unless both the victim's breathing and circulation are supported by mouth-to-mouth ventilation and external chest compression, the brain will die in just a few minutes. Mouth-to-mouth ventilation delivers oxygen to the blood vessels in the lungs whilst external chest compression distributes the oxygenated blood to vital organs including the brain, and the combination of these two procedures is known as cardio-pulmonary resuscitation, or CPR.

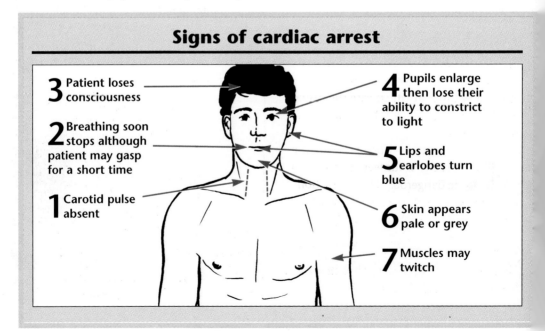

Signs of cardiac arrest

3 Patient loses consciousness

2 Breathing soon stops although patient may gasp for a short time

1 Carotid pulse absent

4 Pupils enlarge then lose their ability to constrict to light

5 Lips and earlobes turn blue

6 Skin appears pale or grey

7 Muscles may twitch

External chest compression

The heart lies between the lungs in the centre of the chest and, if sufficient pressure is repeatedly applied over the breastbone, and then released, blood will flow through the heart and around the body. The reason for performing external chest compression is not to try to restart the heart – this rarely happens without the benefit of a special machine called a defibrillator – but rather to keep the brain supplied with oxygenated blood, until such help can be obtained.

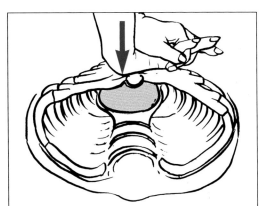

External chest compression maintains the circulation of blood when the heart has stopped beating.

EMERGENCY ACTION

In order to perform external chest compression, the casualty must first be placed on his back on a firm surface. If the patient is in bed, immediately move him onto the floor. External chest compression should only be performed if the heart has stopped beating, in which case the casualty will be unconscious and the carotid pulse will be absent.

It must never be practised on a healthy volunteer as this could be dangerous. The instructions that follow apply only to adults. For the resuscitation of children, see pages 27-31.

1 First establish that the heart has stopped beating by checking that there is no carotid pulse (see page 15). The casualty will be unconscious. Immediately shout for help or telephone 999 for an ambulance. If you have to make the call yourself, try to be back within two or three minutes.

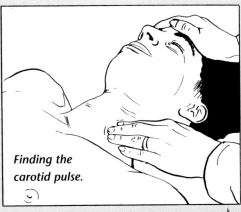

Finding the carotid pulse.

Continued ||||➡

Dealing with an emergency

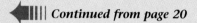

Continued from page 20

2 Kneel beside the casualty's chest and feel for the point where the lower ribs and breastbone meet in the midline. Place your index and middle fingers of one hand (hand A) immediately above this point, then place the heel of your other hand (hand B) directly above these two fingers, in the midline of the chest. Using this method, the heel of hand B should lie along the lower half of the breastbone.

3 Bring hand A up and place it directly on top of hand B, interlocking the fingers; then pull all the fingers away from the chest wall leaving just the heel of the lower hand in contact with the breastbone.

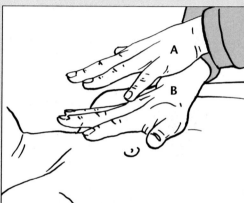

Place hand "A" on top of hand "B" and interlock the fingers, pulling them clear of the chest wall.

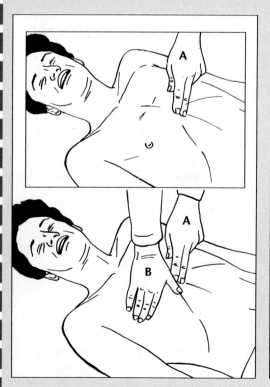

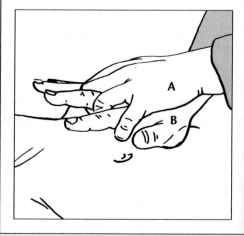

4 Position yourself so that your shoulders are directly over the casualty's chest. With your arms locked straight, rock forward slightly and allow your upper body weight to bear down smoothly on the casualty's breastbone. Aim to depress the chest about 1½ to 2 inches (4 to 5 centimetres), then release the pressure. Keeping your hands in contact with the chest, press straight down again at a rate of around 80 compressions per minute. Try to use a smooth action not a jerky one.

5 To be of any benefit, external chest compressions have to be combined with mouth-to mouth ventilations, so give 15 compressions followed by 2 mouth-to-mouth ventilations, and continue like this as long as necessary. Bear in mind that any serious bleeding may have to be controlled quickly, otherwise there may be insufficient blood left to carry oxygen to the vital organs including the brain (see page 37).

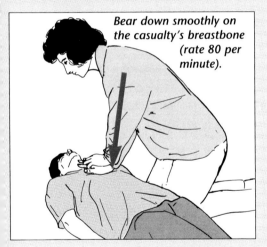

Bear down smoothly on the casualty's breastbone (rate 80 per minute).

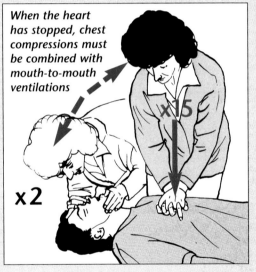

When the heart has stopped, chest compressions must be combined with mouth-to-mouth ventilations

x15

x2

Only stop CPR if:

• Someone is able to take over from you, or
• You are exhausted, or
• You notice an improvement in the casualty's condition (his colour improves, or he starts to move or groan). If this happens, you should immediately check the carotid pulse. If it has returned, and if the casualty is also breathing normally, place him in the recovery position (see page 25-26). If the pulse returns but breathing does not, continue with mouth-to-mouth ventilations at a rate of 10 per minute. Check the carotid pulse at the end of every minute and be prepared to restart full CPR if necessary.

Dealing with an emergency

The recovery position

Although mouth-to-mouth ventilation and external cardiac compression are truly vital skills, it is the ability of the First Aider to establish and maintain an open airway for an unconscious casualty that is the single most important aspect of emergency aid. Turning an unconscious casualty into the recovery position not only pulls the tongue clear of the back of the throat, but also allows any mucus, blood or vomit to drain safely from the mouth.

First treat life-threatening injuries

Once it has been established that the unconscious casualty is breathing adequately and has a pulse, any serious or life-threatening conditions should be treated before the casualty is turned. Bleeding must be stopped by applying local pressure to wounds (see page 37), and fractures should be supported or splinted to prevent further damage (see page 61). Before turning the casualty, remove watches, spectacles or any sharp items of jewellery, and turn the stones of any rings into the palm. Feel the pockets and remove any hard or sharp objects such as loose change and keys.

Which way to turn?

The direction in which a casualty is turned will depend on a number of factors such as the space available/local obstructions, the slope of the ground and any associated injuries. Each case has to be judged on its merits but, as a general rule, it is better to turn the casualty onto his injured side. This is particularly important if chest injuries have been sustained, the good or better side being kept uppermost. Sometimes the unconscious casualty will be discovered already lying on his side. So long as he is breathing adequately and has a pulse, move him as little as possible and make only those minor adjustments necessary to ensure that he has an open airway and is in a stable position.

When neck injuries are suspected

 If you suspect that there may be a neck injury, it is most important that you exercise great care when turning the casualty, to avoid aggravating the injury (see pages 71-73). Try to ensure that the neck is not allowed to twist or to move excessively in any direction and, if possible, have a competent person take responsibility solely for controlling the head and neck as the casualty is turned. Always keep the face and chest pointing in the same direction, and only use the minimum of head tilt necessary to maintain an open airway.

EMERGENCY ACTION

1 With the casualty lying on his back, start by tilting the head backwards in order to open the airway, and then straighten the legs. Now adjust the nearside arm so that the shoulder and elbow joints are at right angles, palm uppermost 'like a policeman on point duty'.

2 Kneeling alongside the casualty, take hold of the far arm and bring it across the chest, pressing the back of this hand into contact with the nearside cheek. Keep hold of the hand as this will enable you to control the head and neck as the casualty is turned.

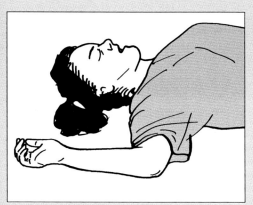

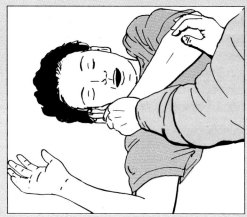

3 With your other hand, reach over the far leg and slide it under the lower thigh. Then lift the leg so that the knee bends to a right angle. Roll the casualty towards you by pulling on the lower thigh whilst controlling the movement of the head and neck with your other hand.

Continued ||||➡

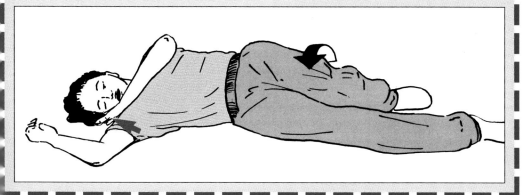

Dealing with an emergency

Continued from page 25

EMERGENCY ACTION

4 Once the casualty is on his side, gently tilt the head back to keep the airway open and use the hand beneath the cheek to maintain this position. Finally make any adjustments to the position of the other limbs to ensure maximum stability and check the respiratory rate and pulse.

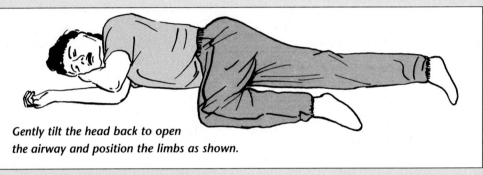

Gently tilt the head back to open the airway and position the limbs as shown.

5 You should try to stay with the casualty until help arrives, keeping a regular check on the breathing and pulse. Should it become necessary to start mouth-to-mouth ventilation or external chest compression, you must first return the casualty onto his back. If you must leave to telephone for an ambulance, first place a rolled-up garment or some other suitable object behind the casualty. This will prevent him rolling onto his back should he partially regain consciousness and begin to move.

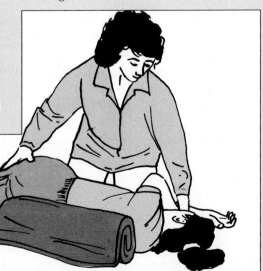

An object placed behind the casualty will increase stability.

Resuscitation of children

Priorities

As far as resuscitation is concerned, the same basic principles apply in children as in adults, and the priorities remain:

 a clear Airway to allow oxygen-containing air to reach the lungs

 adequate Breathing to allow the blood in the lungs to be replenished with oxygen

 an effective Circulation of blood to distribute oxygen round the body.

Because a child's airway is relatively narrow, it can easily become obstructed by a foreign body. Even mild inflammation of the lining of the air passages can narrow them down enough to cause breathing difficulties.

Except following an electric shock, sudden cardiac arrest is a rare event in children. When a child's heart stops beating, this is usually the result of a lack of oxygen for a prolonged period, and explains why the outcome of cardiac arrests in children is often worse than in adults. On the other hand, results of resuscitation of breathing before cardiac arrest has occurred are often excellent, as children are able to tolerate longer periods of oxygen starvation.

Since the great majority of situations requiring resuscitation in children are preventable, time spent learning paediatric CPR techniques is likely to be less productive than time spent preventing those situations arising in the first place.

Study the scene

When dealing with a child who has stopped breathing, the surroundings will often provide a clue as to the nature of the problem. Thus, a toddler found in his cot surrounded by sweets probably has a blocked airway, another lying by a power-point may have received an electric shock, whilst a child found at the foot of a tree is likely to have sustained a head injury.

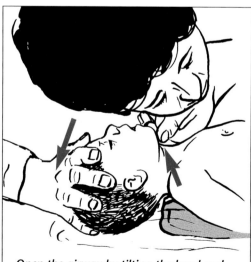

A **Airway**
A child's airway can be opened by tilting the head back and lifting the chin. However, tilting an infant's head too far back can close the airway again, so exaggerated extension of the neck

Open the airway by tilting the head and lifting the chin. Avoid excessive tilt.

Dealing with an emergency

should be avoided. A small folded blanket placed under the child's shoulder blades can help to maintain the correct degree of head tilt. A neutral position is usually best for babies, with the head tilted slightly further back in older children. The bony point of the chin can be lifted with the tips of one or two fingers, but care should be taken to avoid compressing the soft tissues under the chin, as pressure here could actually block the airway.

If there is a strong suspicion that the child is choking, the mouth can be opened and inspected, but only those foreign bodies that can be easily grasped should be removed manually. Finger sweeps should be avoided because of the very real danger of pushing

the obstruction even further down the airway. Babies should immediately be straddled over the rescuer's forearm in a head-down position, and several firm slaps delivered between the shoulder blades. The aim is to expel the foreign body by compressing the chest against the forearm. Under no circumstances should abdominal thrusts be attempted in a child below the age of one year because of the risk of serious injury to abdominal organs.

Older children can be placed head-down across the rescuer's lap whilst back slaps are delivered. Abdominal thrusts should only be attempted if repeated back slaps have failed to relieve the obstruction.

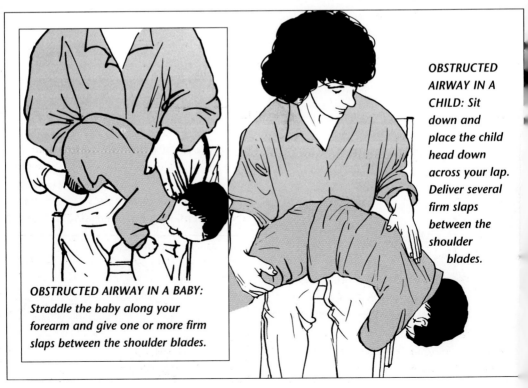

OBSTRUCTED AIRWAY IN A BABY: Straddle the baby along your forearm and give one or more firm slaps between the shoulder blades.

OBSTRUCTED AIRWAY IN A CHILD: Sit down and place the child head down across your lap. Deliver several firm slaps between the shoulder blades.

Breathing

Look, listen and feel for signs of breathing.

- **Look** for rise and fall of the chest.
- **Listen** for the sound of air coming from the mouth.
- **Feel** for the movement of air on your cheek.

If breathing has stopped, first try adjusting the airway by tilting the head a little more, *or a little less*. If there is still no sign of breathing, prepare to give mouth-to-mouth ventilation, or mouth-to-nose-and-mouth ventilation in infants. The force and volume of air used will vary according to the size of the child but should be sufficient to raise the chest. If the chest does not rise easily despite the rescuer adjusting the head tilt, it should be assumed that there is a foreign body blocking the airway and appropriate measures should be taken. Next give 5 breaths each lasting 1-1^1/2 seconds.

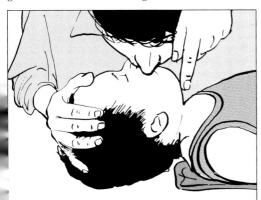

With the airway held open, seal your lips around the baby's nose and mouth, and blow carefully.

Then, providing there is a pulse, the rate of inflation is one every three seconds for infants (20 per minute) or one every four seconds for older children (15 per minute).

Circulation

In an infant (i.e. a child below the age of one year), the upper arm (brachial) pulse should be used to check if the heart is beating. This can be located down the inner aspect of the upper arm between the shoulder and the elbow (where you would find the seam of a jacket sleeve). In older children, the carotid pulse should be used, as in adults.

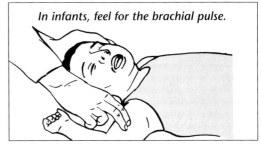

In infants, feel for the brachial pulse.

If the pulse is absent, or is less than 60 beats per minute in an infant below one year old, full cardio-pulmonary resuscitation will be required. To find the correct place to apply external chest compression in infants,

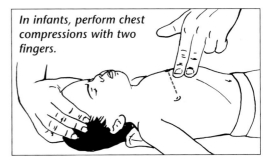

In infants, perform chest compressions with two fingers.

draw an imaginary line between the nipples, and position the tips of two fingers, one finger's-breadth below this line directly over the breastbone.

The breastbone is then depressed with these two fingers to a depth of $1/2$-1 inch (1.5-2.5 cm.), 100 times-a-minute.

In older children, feel for the place where the lower ribs meet at the lower end of the breastbone, and place the heel of one hand, two finger-breadths above this point, directly over the breastbone. Compress with one hand only to a depth of 1-1$1/2$ inches, 100 times-a-minute.

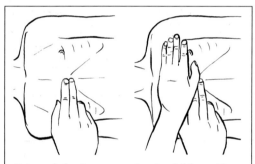

External chest compression in children: Place the heel of one hand two finger-breadths above the point where the lower ribs meet.

In babies, seal your lips around the mouth and nose, and give one mouth-to-nose-and-mouth inflation after every five cardiac compressions. This is most-easily achieved with the infant placed on its back along the rescuer's forearm, with the angle of head tilt controlled by the supporting hand. Infants can be given CPR in this position whilst being transported to a telephone, if no-one else is available to call for an ambulance.

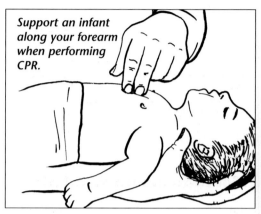

Support an infant along your forearm when performing CPR.

Children below school age are similarly given one inflation for every five cardiac compressions but, because of their larger size, they must be placed on their backs on a firm surface. In larger older children where one-handed chest compression produces insufficient force, use the adult two-handed method with two inflations for every fifteen compressions (compression rate – 80 per minute).

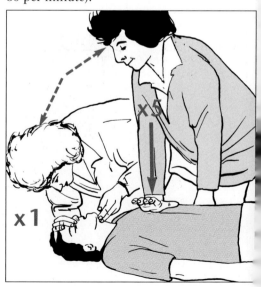

Resuscitation summary

	Infants (below 1yr.)	Children	Adults
Airway			
Finger sweeps	No	No	Yes
Back slaps	Yes	Yes	Yes
Abdominal thrusts	No	Possibly	Yes
Mouth-to-mouth ventilations			
Rate	20 per minute	15 per minute	10 per minute
Chest compressions			
Depth	$1/2$-1″ (1.5-2.5cm)	1-$1^1/2$″ (2.5-4cm)	$1^1/2$-2″ (4-5cm)
Method	2 fingertips	1 hand	2 hands
Rate	100 per minute	100 per minute	80 per minute
CPR ratio			
Compressions to ventilations	5 to 1	5 to 1	15 to 2

CPR in adults
Compression rate = 80 per minute

x15

x2

CPR in children
Compression rate =100 per minute

x5

x1

Part two

The A-Z of first aid

Allergies

The body's immune system protects us from infection by bacteria and viruses. It is primed to recognise our own tissues, so that any invading foreign material can be immediately identified and destroyed. On the whole this arrangement serves us well, but sometimes the immune system reacts inappropriately, causing allergies. Substances capable of causing an allergic reaction are known as allergens.

Allergies often result in nothing worse than an itchy rash, sneezing or mild wheeziness. Mild reactions are best managed by avoiding the allergen if possible, or by treatment with drugs, such as antihistamines. Occasionally, however, a life-threatening allergic reaction called anaphylactic shock can occur.

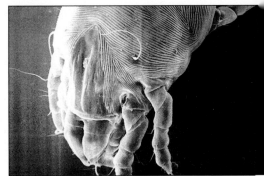

Micrograph of a house dust mite

Allergies can arise after:

● Ingestion of foods like shellfish, strawberries and nuts, or drugs like penicillin and aspirin.
● Inhalation of air-borne particles, such as pollens, dust from feathers and animal hair.
● Absorption of substances through the skin, e.g. nickel salts from cheap jewellery.
● Injection of drugs like penicillin, or a 'natural' injection of bee or wasp venom.

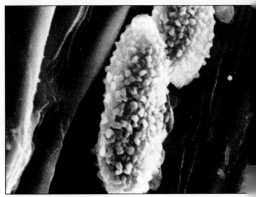

Micrograph of grass pollen grains

Anaphylactic shock

Anaphylactic shock usually follows an injection or sting, and frequently develops within the space of a few minutes. Victims are often aware of their allergy, having had a previous adverse reaction. They may carry a warning card, or wear a warning pendant or bracelet marked 'Medic-Alert' or 'SOS Talisman'. Some may even possess an antidote to be injected in an emergency.

Signs include some or all of the following:

- Widespread, blotchy, raised, itchy, red rash ('hives').
- Swelling of the eyelids, lips, tongue or hands.
- Wheezing and shortness of breath.
- Vomiting and diarrhoea.
- Rapid weak pulse.
- Collapse.

Treatment

1 Help the casualty to lie down and raise the legs to combat shock. Loosen clothing around the neck and chest, and enquire about any known allergies. Keep an eye out for medical warning tags, etc.

2 Dial 999 for an ambulance.

3 If conscious, assist the casualty to take any prescribed medicines or injections.

4 If the casualty becomes unconscious but continues to breathe, turn him into the recovery position (see pages 25-26).

5 Monitor the breathing and pulse, and be prepared to resuscitate if necessary.

Bleeding and shock

The heart

About the size of a clenched fist, the heart is located in the centre of the chest, although it does protrude slightly more to the left side. Its walls consist of strong muscle and, without conscious assistance, the heart beats between 60 and 80 times every minute; a total of over 2,000 million beats in a life-span of 70 years!

The circulation

Our bodies are fuelled by oxygen and all living tissues need a constant supply. Oxygen is picked up in the lungs and is carried around the body attached to a substance called haemoglobin found in red blood cells. Oxygen gets into the tissues by seeping through the walls of tiny blood vessels called capillaries. The right side of the heart receives oxygen-depleted blood from the tissues by way of the veins, and pumps it through the lungs where it is replenished with oxygen. The left side of the heart then takes this oxygenated blood and pumps it back to the tissues by way of the arteries.

Taking a pulse

When taking a pulse, the First Aider should check and record:
- The rate in beats-per-minute (usually done by counting the number of beats over a 15-second period and then multiplying this number by four).
- The strength (does it feel strong or weak?).
- The rhythm (is it regular or irregular?).

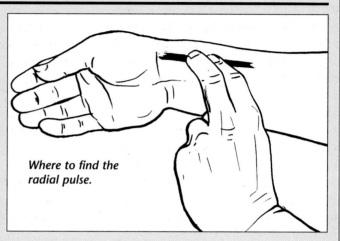

Where to find the radial pulse.

The pulse

Every time the left ventricle contracts, blood is forced along the aorta and into the arteries, and the pressure wave that is generated causes the elastic walls of the arteries to expand briefly. Where arteries run close to the surface, and in particular where they also pass over bone, a pulsation can be detected if the pads on the tips of the fingers are gently pressed over the artery. The thumb should never be used as it has a pulse of its own which may be mistaken for that of the casualty. For ordinary purposes, the most convenient pulse to feel is that of the radial artery which runs down the thumb side of the front of the wrist.

Blood

When blood is saturated with oxygen it becomes bright red in colour (as in the arteries), but as oxygen is released to the tissues it turns progressively darker (as in the veins). In an average adult, there are about 6 litres (10 pints) of blood in the circulation. Just over half of the blood consists of a straw-coloured fluid called plasma, whilst the rest is

Blood characteristics

	Arteries	Veins	Capillaries
Colour of blood	Bright red	Dark red	Fairly bright
Oxygen content of blood	High	Low	Fairly high
Type of bleeding	Spurts in time with pulse	Continuous flow	Oozing

made up of cells: the oxygen-carrying red cells, white cells which fight infection and platelets which help the blood to clot. Each drop of blood contains around 200 million red cells and, with a life of only 30 days, ageing red cells are constantly being replaced by new ones manufactured in the bone marrow.

Shock

By stepping up red cell production in the bone marrow, our bodies can easily cope with the loss of small quantities of blood. Healthy people can even lose 500 ml at a time - the quantity given by blood donors – with no ill effects. But the loss of a litre or more over a short period is liable to lead to a serious condition called shock. Shock can be defined as a critical loss of circulating blood volume, the remaining volume being unable to meet the needs of the tissues. It arises if large quantities of fluid are lost from the circulation for whatever reason.

Emotional shock

The term 'shock' is commonly used to describe the emotional distress experienced when someone witnesses a frightening event or receives bad news, but this type of emotional shock must not be confused with medical shock which is a life-threatening condition.

When about half the blood volume is lost, the pulse at the wrist disappears and it becomes necessary to feel for the carotid pulse in the neck (see page 15). If shock is allowed to progress, the casualty will lapse into unconsciousness and the heart will eventually stop, so prompt First Aid treatment of bleeding is essential.

How nature controls bleeding

When a blood vessel is damaged its walls contract to reduce the blood flow, whilst tiny blood particles called platelets are attracted to the site of the injury. They set up a local reaction and strands of a special protein called fibrin form and attempt to attach themselves to the vessel wall. More platelets become entangled in the strands of fibrin as the resulting blood clot attempts to plug the leak. Normally the process takes only a few minutes, but if the hole in the vessel wall is large and the blood escapes too rapidly, nature is unable to stem the flow in time to prevent shock. Bleeding may either be internal, where it is retained within the body, or external, where blood escapes from a wound in the skin.

Internal bleeding

Serious internal bleeding can occur when large bones like the pelvis or thigh bone (femur) are fractured, or when abdominal organs like the spleen are damaged. A bleeding stomach ulcer or the rupture of an ectopic pregnancy can also lead to heavy

The causes of shock

- Bleeding.
- Burns.
- Severe diarrhoea and vomiting.
- Serious allergic reactions.
- Heart attack.
- Overwhelming infections etc.

The A-Z of first aid

Symptoms and signs of shock

Symptom or sign	Reason
Skin pale, cool and clammy	Blood vessels in the skin shut down in order to divert their contents to vital organs like the brain and kidneys. Sweat glands are also stimulated.
Pulse rapid	The heart attempts to compensate for a reduction in blood volume by speeding up the circulation.
Pulse weak	The reduction in blood volume causes the blood pressure to fall.
Muscular weakness	There is a reduced supply of blood to the muscles.
Breathing rapid and shallow (known as 'air hunger')	The body tries to get as much oxygen as possible into the limited blood volume.
Nausea and vomiting	Probably a primitive reflex to expel any poisons from the stomach.
Thirst	The brain senses that the body needs more fluid.
Dizziness and deterioration in the level of consciousness	The blood supply to the brain is reduced.

internal bleeding, and the First Aider should always be alert for the symptoms and signs of shock.

External bleeding

External bleeding is easier to diagnose, but accurate estimation of the volume lost can be difficult; a small amount of blood goes a long way on a tiled floor, whereas large quantities can soak into soil leaving hardly a trace. However, if the pulse rate exceeds 100 beats-per-minute, the casualty has probably lost at least 25 per cent of his total blood volume and is in urgent need of treatment. The First Aid treatment of external bleeding is to prevent shock by stopping (or at least slowing down) blood loss to allow the natural clotting process to seal off the injury. External bleeding can nearly always be stopped by applying pressure directly over a wound and elevating the injured part if this is possible.

EMERGENCY ACTION

Large wounds

1 Expose the wound and quickly inspect for embedded glass or other sharp objects (see page 38). If none is seen, apply direct pressure over the wound, or push the edges of a long wound together.

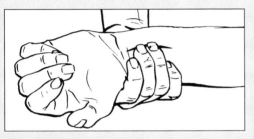

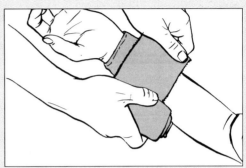

2 Lie the casualty down and elevate the injured part. Continue to apply direct pressure using any convenient

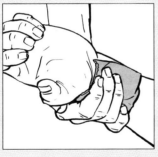

piece of material, e.g. a clean handkerchief, but, ideally, a sterile gauze pad that completely covers the wound.

3 Keep applying direct pressure for at least 5 minutes (10 minutes for arterial bleeding).

4 Secure the pad by means of a firmly applied crêpe bandage - or improvise with a stocking, belt, tie or scarf.

5 If blood soaks through the dressing, DO NOT REMOVE IT. Place another dressing on top and re-bandage firmly.

6 Obtain medical assistance as stitches may be required. Be alert for signs of shock and treat by elevating the casualty's legs.

Recommended items
- Sterile gauze pad.
- Crêpe bandage.
- Safety pins or tape.

IMPORTANT
- Don't waste time washing your hands if the bleeding is heavy; act immediately to prevent shock.
- DO NOT elevate a limb if you suspect it may be fractured.
- NEVER apply a tourniquet.
- Bandage tightly enough to control bleeding but not too tightly. Loosen if numbness or tingling develop, or the limb appears white.

EMERGENCY ACTION
Wounds containing embedded objects

1 Lie the casualty down and expose the wound. Immediately control bleeding by elevating the limb and pressing the edges of the wound against the base of the embedded object.

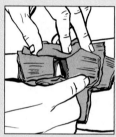

2 Using sterile gauze swabs (or pads of any suitable material) build up a protective ring around the base of the object, until the ring is taller than the object itself.

3 Starting on the side of the object furthest from the heart, bandage firmly over the protective ring, avoiding the embedded object.

4 After one or two turns, pass diagonally beneath the limb and bandage firmly over the protective ring on the opposite side

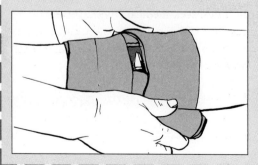

of the object. Continue bandaging alternately above and below (but never directly over) the object, and secure the end.

5 Finish by covering loosely with a sterile gauze dressing (or any clean material) and secure with safety pins or tape.

6 Support and immobilize the injured part in an elevated position and obtain immediate medical assistance.

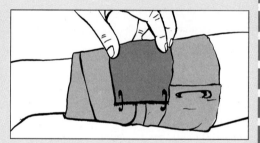

Recommended items
- Sterile gauze dressings.
- Crepe bandage.
- Safety pins or tape.

IMPORTANT
- NEVER attempt to pick out an embedded object from a wound. You could easily worsen the injury and aggravate bleeding. However, if the object appears to be loose, you could attempt to flush it out of the wound with running water.
- If the object is particularly large, leave it protruding through the centre of the protective gauze ring.

Breathing problems

Asthma

Asthma is a common, yet potentially serious, breathing disorder caused by spasm of the muscle found in the walls of the air passages. Sufferers usually experience attacks of wheezing (a high-pitched whistle as they breathe out), together with shortness of breath. The condition is often inherited, and there may be a family history of asthma, eczema, hay fever or urticaria (nettle rash or hives). Allergy to things such as animal hair,

pollen and the house dust mite is sometimes the cause, but attacks of asthma may also be precipitated by:

- Air pollution, including cigarette smoke.
- Exercise, particularly in cold weather.
- Emotion.
- Virus infections of the respiratory tract.

Carbon monoxide poisoning

Carbon monoxide is a colourless, tasteless,

continued on page 41

Treatment of an asthma attack

1 Sit the casualty down and try to reassure and calm him. Allow him to lean forward keeping a straight back, and to rest his arms on a firm surface like a

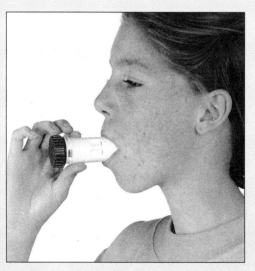

table top. Loosen any tight clothing around the neck and chest, then open a window (but not if the weather is cold).

2 Assist the casualty to take any prescribed medicines such as inhalers, but take care to avoid overdosing, as he may have tried them already. If no medication is available, try giving sips of warm, strong coffee.

3 Inhalers usually work quickly, so if there is no improvement within 15 minutes, seek medical advice. If the casualty starts to go blue around the lips, or becomes confused and drowsy, dial 999 for an ambulance.

4 Whilst awaiting the ambulance, monitor the breathing and pulse and be prepared to resuscitate if necessary (see pages 17-23).

The A-Z of first aid

Chest injuries

Fractured ribs can seriously interfere with breathing, or may cause a lung to collapse. After any chest injury, if breathing appears to be inadequate, you should obtain immediate assistance.

Treatment of a penetrating chest wound

1 Immediately seal the wound with the palm of your hand, or with the casualty's own hand if he is still conscious.

2 Place a sterile dressing or clean pad over the wound, followed by a larger sheet of polythene, clingfilm or similar airtight material, taping the edges securely to the skin on three sides only.

3 Dial 999 for an ambulance.

4 Whilst awaiting the ambulance, monitor the breathing and pulse and be prepared to resuscitate if necessary (see pages 17-23).

5 If the casualty becomes unconscious but continues to breathe, turn him into the recovery position (see pages 25-26), placing him on his **injured** side, and continue to monitor his breathing and pulse.

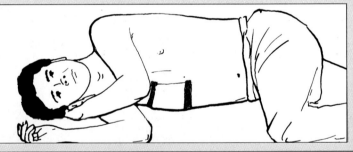

If he is breathing, turn an unconscious casualty onto his injured side.

Treatment of carbon monoxide poisoning

1 Immediately evacuate the casualty into the fresh air. You are unlikely to come to any harm yourself during a brief excursion into a fume-filled garage.

2 Check the casualty's level of consciousness, breathing and pulse, and resuscitate if necessary (see pages 17-23).

3 If the casualty is unconscious but is breathing adequately, turn him into the recovery position (see pages 25-26), then dial 999 for an ambulance.

4 Whilst awaiting the ambulance continue to monitor the breathing and pulse.

continued from page 39
odourless gas that is very toxic when inhaled. Once in the bloodstream, it combines with the haemoglobin in red blood cells, steadily blocking their ability to take up oxygen. If a build up of carbon monoxide is allowed to continue, the brain will eventually die from lack of oxygen. Blood that is saturated with carbon monoxide takes on a cherry-red colour, very obvious in pale-skinned victims of poisoning. Carbon monoxide is a constituent of car exhaust fumes, which is produced when any hydrocarbon fuel burns incompletely, so it is vitally important that appliances such as gas-fired domestic boilers receive adequate ventilation.

Croup

Croup is a common winter-time disorder in children below school age, and is caused by inflammation and swelling of the tissues lining the upper part of the airway. At bedtime the child is usually quite well, but then awakes during the evening with a

Treatment of croup

Even though you may be frightened yourself, try to reassure and calm the child, as panic will only aggravate the breathing difficulties.

1 Generate steam by running a hot bath or boiling a kettle, and sit in the atmosphere with the child upright on your knee.

2 If the attack is severe, and the child starts to turn blue around the lips, dial 999 for an ambulance.

3 If the child stops breathing, immediately try back slaps (see page 28), followed, if necessary by abdominal thrusts in children over the age of 1 year in order to exclude an inhaled foreign body, but **never** attempt blind finger sweeps as this may drastically worsen the obstruction. Mouth-to-mouth ventilation can be tried, but may be ineffective in view of the nature of the problem.

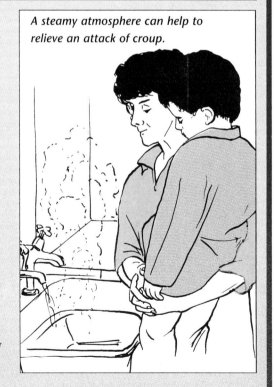

A steamy atmosphere can help to relieve an attack of croup.

The A-Z of first aid

harsh, barking cough and difficulty in breathing. As the child breathes in, there may be a coarse, whistling noise (stridor), and attacks can be frightening for both child and parent.

Most attacks settle within a few hours, but may recur with decreasing severity on subsequent evenings. Occasionally, however, a flap of tissue called the epiglottis becomes involved, threatening to completely block the airway. Epiglottitis tends to affect slightly older children (aged 3 to 6 years), but should be suspected in any child if, in addition to those breathing difficulties already described, there is a high temperature, drooling and pain on swallowing. Epiglottitis is a medical emergency, and the family doctor or an ambulance should be summoned immediately if this condition is suspected.

Smoke inhalation

Fires can produce dense, choking fumes, making breathing impossible. Around 600 people die in fires each year in Britain, and the majority of these deaths are due to smoke inhalation rather than burns. The installation of smoke detectors in all homes could prevent many of these tragedies.

Treatment of smoke inhalation

1 First ensure your own safety. Do not enter buildings that are burning fiercely, or where there are dense fumes. Would-be rescuers can be overcome by smoke in a matter of seconds.

2 After moving the casualty to safety, extinguish clothing that may be alight.

3 Check the casualty's level of consciousness, breathing and pulse, and be prepared to resuscitate if necessary (see pages 17-23).

4 If necessary, treat for burns (see page 45) and shock.

5 All victims of smoke inhalation must be sent to hospital, as serious breathing problems may suddenly arise a number of hours after the incident.

Burns

Causes

Burns are tissue injuries that are commonly, but not exclusively, caused by heat. They arise as a result of exposure to:

1 **Extremes of temperature.**
Both high and low temperatures can cause burns. High-temperature burns can be caused by dry heat, e.g. a flame or hot object or friction, or wet heat, e.g. a hot liquid or steam. Very cold substances will also damage tissues, and liquid nitrogen and solid carbon dioxide (dry ice) are sometimes used by doctors to burn away verrucas and warts.

Depth of burns

The severity of any burn will depend on its type, depth, size and location. Burns to the skin may be superficial, intermediate (partial-thickness burns) or deep (full-thickness burns).

Type	Appearance	Pain	Scarring	Notes
Superficial	Redness of the skin	Yes, of variable intensity	No	e.g. mild sunburn or slight scald. Medical attention unnecessary unless extensive
Intermediate	Blister formation with a moist, raw surface beneath and marked local swelling	Yes, frequently severe	Possibly	Seek medical advice if area larger than a 50p. coin. Can prove fatal if more than 50% of body involved. Can become infected
Deep	Charred, grey or waxy-looking surface	No, except possibly at margins	Yes	Nerve endings also destroyed, hence lack of pain. Skin graft sometimes required. Always seek medical advice

2 Corrosive chemicals.
Strong acids, such as sulphuric acid found in car batteries, or strong alkalis found in proprietary oven cleaners, can cause burns on contact.

3 Radiation.
Ordinary sunburn is an example of a radiation burn.

4 Electricity.
Electrical burns are often more serious than at first they appear. The only visible damage

For chemical burns to the eyes, immediately wash with water under a running cold water tap or by pouring water from a jug and then seek hospital treatment immediately

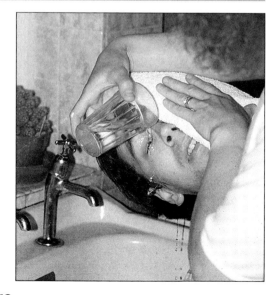

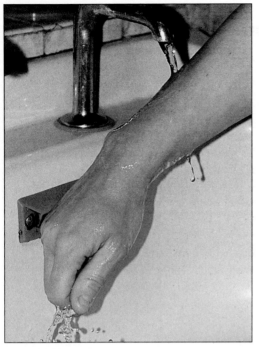

Hold the burn under cold running water for ten minutes. This will minimize tissue damage and greatly reduce pain.

may be burns to the skin at the current's entry and exit points, but very high temperatures can be generated as electrical energy passes through the body, and serious damage can be inflicted to deep tissues such as blood vessels, muscle and bone.

Be aware that an electric shock may cause the casualty's heart to stop beating, so cardio-pulmonary resuscitation may be required.

⚠️ **Important** – Do not touch the casualty's skin if he is still in contact with the current. Where high voltage currents are involved, do not approach within 18 metres of the casualty (see pages 54-55).

Area of burn

The area of a burn can be quickly estimated by employing the so-called, 'Rule of Nines', in which specific regions of the body are regarded as representing nine per cent, or multiples of nine per cent of the total surface area. Even superficial burns, if they affect more than nine per cent of the body, will require medical attention. Using the Rule of Nines, the area of a burn is calculated as follows:

Area of burns on the body

Region	Area
Head	1 x 9%
Left Arm	1 x 9%
Right arm	1 x 9%
Front of torso	2 x 9%
Back of torso	2 x 9%
Left leg	2 x 9%
Right leg	2 x 9%
Genital area	1%
Total	**100%**

Treatment of burns to the skin

1 Ensure your own safety.
Do not endanger your own life by entering burning buildings to rescue others – call the Fire Service. Apart from the danger of burns, you risk death or injury from falling masonry and smoke inhalation.

With chemical burns, avoid self-contamination by wearing protective gloves.

If the casualty has sustained electrical burns, first ensure that the current has been switched off.

2 Extinguish any flames.
If a casualty's clothing is alight, make him lie down and douse him with cold water to extinguish the flames, but DO NOT use water if he is in contact with a live electrical source.

Alternatively, smother the flames with a rug or any other suitable material, but avoid synthetic fabrics which can melt and cause serious burns in their own right, and do not roll the casualty.

3 Cool rapidly.
Immediately hold the burn under cold running water for ten minutes. This will minimize tissue damage and greatly reduce pain.

Irrigation will wash away and dilute corrosive chemicals, but burns caused by caustic alkalis may require treatment for up to twenty minutes.

4 Anticipate swelling.
Any jewellery, such as rings, bracelets and watches, should be removed to prevent them constricting swollen tissues.

Elevating an affected limb will help to minimize any swelling.

5 Cover the burns.
Burns should be covered to help prevent infection. Ideally a non-stick, sterile dressing should be used but, in an emergency, a clean linen sheet or pillowcase cut to size will do. Alternatively, use kitchen clingfilm which allows the burns to be inspected by doctors without the need to first remove the dressing. For burns to hands and feet, place them in a clear plastic bag.

Under no circumstances should you apply creams, ointments, sprays, butter, oil or fat to burns. At best they do no good, and hospital staff will only have to remove them, resulting in unnecessary extra pain for the casualty.

Do not use adhesive dressings on burns. Do not deliberately burst or prick any blisters, as you could introduce infection.

6 Conserve body heat.
Once treatment is complete, cover the patient with blankets if the burns are extensive, as a sudden drop in body temperature (hypothermia) can occur.

If necessary, treat for shock by elevating the casualty's legs and arrange transfer to hospital.

The A-Z of first aid

Choking

At the upper level of the voice box (larynx), the throat divides into two passages; the oesophagus (gullet) behind, and the trachea (windpipe) in front. The oesophagus conveys food to the stomach whilst the trachea leads down to the lungs. Each time we swallow, a flap of cartilage called the epiglottis moves down to prevent food or drink entering the air passages. Choking occurs when any foreign object becomes lodged in the airway: a common cause of accidental death, particularly in children.

During a choking attack, the obstruction may be one of the following:

● Complete: in which case breathing ceases and the casualty soon becomes unconscious.
● Partial: where the casualty continues to breathe, albeit noisily and with difficulty, and may or may not lose consciousness.

In a choking emergency there is no time to call for professional assistance. With the airway blocked, brain damage will begin within three or four minutes from lack of oxygen. In less than ten minutes the brain will be completely destroyed with no hope of recovery.

Features of a choking attack

Choking may occur when someone suddenly laughs or goes to sneeze whilst food is in the mouth. Children who mouth small toys, food or sweets whilst running and playing are also at risk. A typical victim with complete obstruction of the airway will:

1 Immediately bring his hand up to his throat, with thumb and index finger spread widely into a 'V' – a very characteristic sign.
2 Show signs of acute distress or panic.
3 Be unable to speak or breathe.
4 Become unconscious after a short period.

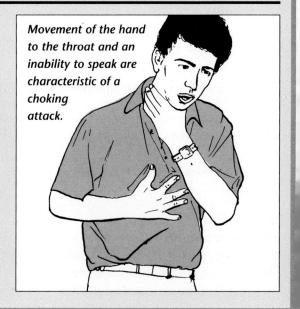

Movement of the hand to the throat and an inability to speak are characteristic of a choking attack.

EMERGENCY ACTION

The movement of the hand to the throat and the inability to speak are so typical of a choking attack that, should these signs be present, the First Aider should immediately suspect a blocked airway. Do not wait for the casualty to become unconscious, act immediately.

1 Ask the casualty, 'Are you choking?' Although unable to speak, he will usually nod his head in reply.

2 If the obstruction is only partial and noisy breathing is still present, encourage the casualty to breathe in slowly and deeply, then to cough forcefully. It will help to bend the casualty forward over a chair back and to give up to five firm slaps between the shoulder blades followed by finger sweeps.

3 If the airway obstruction is complete, or an incomplete obstruction is not cleared by coughing or back slaps, immediately perform abdominal thrusts, otherwise known as the Heimlich manoeuvre, but abdominal thrusts and finger sweeps should NOT be used in

infants (for instructions on clearing an infant's airway, see page 28).

Abdominal thrusts

When abdominal thrusts are performed, the casualty's diaphragm is forced upwards, and the accompanying sudden increase in pressure within the lungs and air passages creates an artificial cough. This often succeeds in expelling the obstruction, like a cork from a popgun.

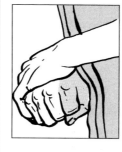

The thumb and index finger form a knob (shaded) which is placed against the abdomen slightly above the navel.

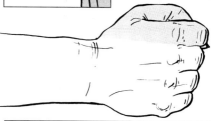

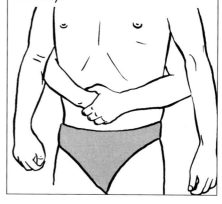

Abdominal thrusts can be performed from behind on a standing or sitting casualty.

The A-Z of first aid

Treatment of choking (casualty conscious)

1 Position yourself behind the casualty and encircle your arms around his waist.

2 With one hand, make a fist and place the thumb against the casualty's abdomen just above the tummy button, but well below the bottom of the breastbone.

3 With your free hand, grasp this fist and pull it into the casualty's abdomen using a quick and forceful upward thrust.

4 Repeat the thrust as many as six times, if necessary, in order to clear the airway.

5 If the casualty becomes unconscious, proceed as below.

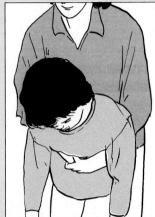

Pull your fist into the casualty's abdomen using a quick and forceful upward thrust.

Treatment of choking (casualty unconscious)

1 After shouting for help, quickly place the casualty on his back and kneel astride his hips, facing his head.

2 Place the heel of one hand on the abdomen, slightly above the tummy button with the fingertips just below the ribcage.

3 Put your other hand on top and deliver one or more quick upward thrusts until the obstruction is expelled, carefully picking out any object that appears in the mouth.

4 If the casualty starts to breathe but remains unconscious, place him in the recovery position (see pages 25-26)

5 If the casualty does not start to breathe immediately, first check the carotid pulse (see page 15).

6 If a pulse is present, give ten mouth to mouth inflations over a period of one minute (one breath every six seconds). If breathing hasn't returned after one minute, send a bystander, or go yourself, to dial 999 for an ambulance. If you have to leave to telephone for help, try to return within two or three minutes, then continue ventilating at a rate of one breath every six seconds, until breathing returns. Check the carotid pulse at the end of every minute and be prepared to perform full CPR if necessary (see pages 17-23).

7 If the pulse and breathing are absent, first send a bystander or go yourself to dial 999 for an ambulance. Then give repeated cycles of two mouth-to-mouth ventilations followed by fifteen external chest compressions, until help arrives.

Treating choking on a child

Abdominal thrusts should NOT be performed on infants below the age of one year, because of the risk of damage to abdominal organs. Neither should blind finger sweeps be attempted. Instead, modified back slaps are recommended (see page 28). In older children, abdominal thrusts can be administered either from behind, or with the child lying on its back, but less force should be used than in adults.

Treatment of choking (pregnant casualty)

Abdominal thrusts can safely be used to clear an airway obstruction during the first six months of pregnancy. However, in advanced pregnancy, there may be insufficient space between the lower border of the ribcage and the enlarging womb to allow a thrust to be delivered here. As an alternative, chest thrusts can be administered from behind in the form of repeated, sharp 'bear hugs'.

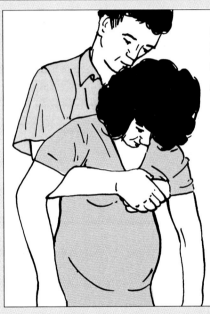

Chest thrusts can be used in advanced pregnancy.

Treatment of choking (self-treatment)

You can even use abdominal thrusts on yourself, should you ever suffer a choking attack. This can be done by placing a fist slightly above the tummy button and below the ribcage, grasping this fist with your other hand and pulling it into your abdomen with a quick upward thrust. Alternatively, you can position yourself over a fixed object like a chair back or table edge, ramming your upper abdomen against the object to deliver a quick upward thrust, and repeating if necessary.

The A-Z of first aid

Diabetes

What is diabetes?

The cells of our bodies get their energy by breaking down a sugar called glucose, in the presence of oxygen, and a lack of either of these basic substances can do serious damage, particularly to the brain. Oxygen is absorbed during respiration, and glucose is obtained from eating sugars and starchy foods, collectively known as carbohydrates. Once digested, carbohydrates are broken down by the liver into glucose.

Sugar diabetes, or diabetes mellitus, is the disease that arises when the pancreas fails to produce sufficient quantities of a hormone called insulin. Insulin acts as a kind of chemical key that unlocks the cells of the body, enabling them to take up glucose. Without insulin, cells would die from lack of glucose, despite the presence of high levels in the bloodstream. Symptoms of diabetes include thirst, weakness, tiredness, weight loss and the passing of large quantities of urine. Severe diabetes can progress to coma and death, if left untreated.

Treatment of diabetes

Mild diabetes often responds to a simple restriction of dietary carbohydrate intake. A moderate form of the disease will sometimes respond to tablets called hypoglycaemic agents, which act partly by stimulating natural insulin secretion, and partly by mimicking insulin and persuading cells to take up some of the available glucose. Severe forms require treatment with insulin, which has to be given by injection because it would be broken down and inactivated if taken by mouth. To keep blood sugar levels stable, an insulin-dependent diabetic must balance the insulin dose against both his carbohydrate intake and energy requirements.

Diabetic emergencies

There are two types of diabetic emergency which can result in unconsciousness - hypoglycaemia (too little glucose in the blood), and hyperglycaemia (too much glucose in the blood).

First Aid treatment for diabetic emergencies

Diabetics suffering from hyperglycaemia (high blood sugar levels) should be transferred to hospital for treatment, whereas those with hypoglycaemia (low blood sugar levels) need immediate treatment to minimize the risk of brain damage. Consult the table on page 51, and if you are still not sure which type of diabetic emergency you are dealing with, treat the casualty for a low blood sugar as extra sugar will do little immediate harm even if the blood sugar levels are high.

Hypoglycaemia

Hypoglycaemia usually comes on suddenly, and arises when a diabetic:

● Takes too much insulin (or accidentally injects the insulin directly into the bloodstream), causing a sudden fall in the blood glucose level.

● Fails to eat enough, and so fails to replenish the glucose levels in the blood.

● Takes too much exercise, burning up the available glucose.

Hyperglycaemia

Hyperglycaemia usually comes on gradually over a period of hours or days.
It occurs in:

● New diabetics before diagnosis.

● Known diabetics on inadequate treatment.

● Diabetics who develop other illnesses which upset control of their disease.

Distinguishing between hypoglycaemia and hyperglycaemia

	Hypoglycaemia (low blood glucose)	Hyperglycaemia (high blood glucose)
History		
Onset	Rapid (minutes)	Gradual (hours or days)
Inadequate food intake	Yes	No
Insulin dose	In excess of requirements	Inadequate (or not taking)
Strenuous exercise	Often	Rare
Symptoms		
	Dizziness, headache, and hunger	Abdominal pain, nausea, thirst and vomiting
Signs		
Behaviour	Confused, staggering, and possibly aggressive	Restless
Breath	Normal	Sweet and fruity like nail varnish or pear drops
Breathing	Normal or shallow	Rapid and deep
Response to sugar	Rapid (1 or 2 minutes)	None
Shaking or fits	When blood sugar very low	Rare
Skin	Pale, cool and moist	Flushed, warm and dry

EMERGENCY ACTION

Hypoglycaemia (low blood glucose)

This occurs when an insulin-dependent diabetic has taken too much insulin, has eaten insufficient food or has performed strenuous exercise.

Diabetics offer carry a warning card, or they may wear a bracelet or pendant marked 'Medic-Alert' or 'SOS Talisman'. Amongst their possessions you may also find sugar lumps or an insulin syringe.

1 If the casualty is conscious, help him to sit or lie down, and give sugar by mouth in the form of a sweet drink or sugar cubes (two cubes are usually sufficient).

2 If the casualty is semi-conscious or unco-operative, you can try carefully smearing a small quantity of honey or syrup onto the lining of the cheek.

3 If unconscious, open the airway, check the breathing and pulse, and resuscitate if necessary (see pages 17-23). If breathing, turn into the recovery position (see pages 25-26), then dial 999 for an ambulance.

Recommended items

● Sweet drinks or sugar cubes.
(Note: Artificial sweeteners are not effective.)

IMPORTANT

● DO NOT attempt to give an unconscious casualty anything by mouth.
● If there is no improvement within 5 minutes of administering sugar, dial 999 for an ambulance.

Drowning

Drowning is a common cause of accidental death, particularly amongst young children. In some countries it is the commonest cause of death between the ages of one and four years and, for every death, it is estimated that there are between six and ten cases of near-drowning requiring admission to hospital. Most of these accidents could probably be avoided if all children were taught to swim at an early age, and domestic swimming pools and ponds were always fenced off.

The process of drowning

A drowning person often lacks the energy to shout, but may attempt to signal to onlookers, so the sight of a waving swimmer should always raise suspicion. Once submerged, the victim is eventually unable to resist taking a breath, allowing water to enter the upper airway. This immediately causes muscular spasm in the throat impeding breathing. Consciousness is then quickly lost as the oxygen supply to the brain falls. Often only small amounts of water enter the lungs, compared with the large quantities that tend to be swallowed. The latter presents an extra hazard, as casualties frequently vomit whilst being resuscitated. Resuscitation is also complicated by the fact that the lungs may become stiff, making them difficult to inflate.

Immersion in cold water

Under normal circumstances, the brain will start to suffer permanent damage if deprived of oxygen for as little as three or four minutes. However, when the water is cold, and particularly where young children are concerned, survival times may be much greater as the body uses up less oxygen at low temperatures and recovery from submersion in icy water for periods of thirty minutes and longer, is not uncommon in children. In view of this, it is always worth attempting to resuscitate children involved in drowning accidents, even when they have been submerged for lengthy periods.

Rescue from drowning

1 First ensure your own safety. Do not enter very cold, deep water, or places where there are strong currents. If possible, throw a buoyancy aid or rope to someone in difficulties, or pull them to land with the aid of a branch or stick. When carrying a casualty out of water, keep his head low to encourage water to drain from the upper airway, and also to minimize the risk of inhalation of vomit.

2 If the ground slopes, position the casualty with his head lowermost and try to keep him warm.

3 If the casualty is unconscious, shout for help, then open the airway and **look**, **listen** and **feel** for signs of breathing (see page 14).

4 If breathing is absent, check the carotid pulse (see page 15), then quickly inspect inside the mouth for weeds or other obstructions. If necessary, clear the airway by performing finger sweeps (see page 13) except in small children, or abdominal thrusts (see page 19) except in infants below the age of one year (see page 28). Do not waste time trying to drain water from the lungs as this is unnecessary.

5 If the casualty is not breathing but the carotid pulse is present, perform mouth-to-mouth ventilation (see pages 17-18).

6 If breathing and pulse are absent, first send a bystander, or go yourself, to dial 999 for an ambulance. Then give full cardio-pulmonary resuscitation until help arrives (see pages 22-23).

7 Ensure that all victims of near-drowning are taken to hospital, as serious breathing problems can develop many hours after an apparent full recovery.

The A-Z of first aid

Electrical injuries

The passage of an electrical current through the body can result in:

- **Burns** Electricity can cause severe burns to deep tissues.
- **Cardiac arrest** An electric shock can cause the heart to go into spasm (ventricular fibrillation) and stop beating. Once ventricular fibrillation has become established, the heartbeat can only be restored with the aid of a special machine called a defibrillator, carried on most emergency ambulances. Until the ambulance arrives, the First Aider's task is to keep the casualty's brain supplied with oxygen by performing cardio-pulmonary resuscitation.
- **Associated problems** An electric shock can also produce sudden contraction of voluntary muscles, causing the casualty to be propelled some distance. As a result, fractures

and other injuries may be sustained. Muscular spasm can prevent the casualty releasing his grip on the electrical source, when breathing may be interrupted due to spasm of the breathing muscles.

Lightning

A direct lightning strike can result in instantaneous death and severe burns. During a thunder storm, the risks of being struck are significantly increased by sheltering under a tall tree, or by being caught in an exposed setting such as a golf course. Those who survive may require treatment for burns (see page 45), and it is worth noting that it is safe to handle all victims immediately, as their bodies do not retain any charge. Amongst survivors, temporary psychological disturbances are common.

High-voltage shocks

High-voltage shocks from overhead power lines or electrical transformers are likely to prove fatal, and severe burns are often sustained. When dealing with an incident involving a high-voltage current:

1 Call the emergency services.

2 Keep away and keep others away from the scene until an official from the electricity company confirms that the current has been switched off.

⚠ Be aware that high-voltage electricity can jump ('arc') across gaps as wide as 18 metres (20 yards), killing anyone who approaches. If power lines are downed in an road accident, shout to vehicle occupants to stay put.

3 When you are told it is safe to approach, assess the casualty's level of consciousness and follow the ABC of resuscitation (see pages 17-23).

4 Treat for burns (see page 45) and shock.

Low-voltage shocks

⚠️ IMPORTANT - Do not touch the casualty's skin if he is still in contact with the current.

1 First turn off the current by unplugging, removing a fuse or switching off at the mains. If this is not possible, stand on any dry, insulating material like a rubber mat, telephone directory or thick pile of newspapers, and separate the casualty and the electrical source by means of a wooden chair, broom or walking stick. Alternatively, wear rubber gloves and carefully tug at dry clothing.

2 As soon as it is safe, assess the casualty's level of consciousness, breathing and pulse, then follow the **ABC** of resuscitation if necessary (see pages 17-23).

3 Treat any burns by cooling with water (see page 45), but take care not to put yourself at risk of electric shock.

4 If necessary, treat for shock by elevating the legs.

5 Arrange for removal to hospital unless there are obviously no injuries.

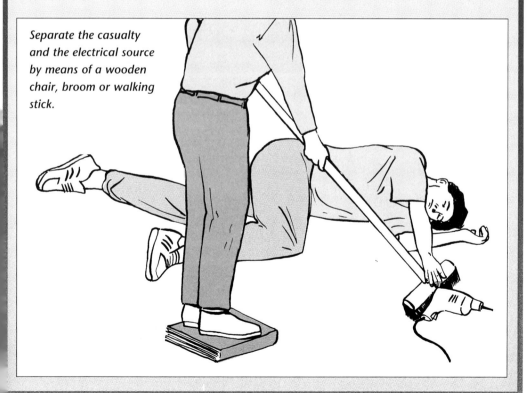

Separate the casualty and the electrical source by means of a wooden chair, broom or walking stick.

The A-Z of first aid

Fits, faints and funny turns

Epilepsy

Epileptic fits, sometimes referred to as seizures or convulsions, occur when there is a sudden eruption of abnormal electrical activity in the brain. Petit mal epilepsy is a minor form of the disease which may cause nothing more than a momentary lapse in concentration, but the major form, called grand mal epilepsy, results in sudden loss of consciousness and violent jerking of the body and limbs. Although major attacks can be frightening to observe, they rarely last for more than a few minutes, and the main problem may be injuries sustained in the fall. Some sufferers experience strange sensations warning of an impending attack, a phenomenon called the aura.

Features of a major fit

- The casualty suddenly loses consciousness and falls to the ground, often emitting a strange cry.
- The muscles become rigid, causing the back to arch and the limbs to flex (tonic phase).
- Breathing stops, and the face and neck become purple and congested.
- Jerky movements of the whole body then begin, and there is a return to noisy breathing through a clenched jaw. Frothing at the mouth, tongue biting and incontinence of urine are common at this stage of the fit (clonic phase).
- Usually within a minute, the muscles start to relax and breathing becomes quieter, although the casualty may remain unconscious for several more minutes.
- On regaining consciousness, the casualty may be confused or act strangely or even violently for a while.

Fainting

A faint is a period of impaired consciousness resulting from a temporary reduction in the

---

Treatment of a major fit

1 If you notice someone about to have a fit, help him to fall safely and place him on his back.

2 Clear a space around the casualty and put some padding under his head.

3 Loosen any tight clothing around the neck and chest. The discovery of an epilepsy warning card might tell you about the likely pattern of the attack.

4 Do not attempt to restrain the casualty, and never put anything in his mouth.

5 As the attack begins to subside, get ready to place the casualty in the recovery position (see pages 25-26) as soon as all jerky movements have stopped.

6 Treat any injuries sustained during the attack.

7 If the casualty has not regained consciousness within 15 minutes, dial 999 for an ambulance.

blood supply to the brain. Fainting is caused by a reflex mechanism which slows the heart and allows blood to pool in the vessels of the lower limbs, reducing the supply available to the brain. An attack can be brought on by pain and emotion, or by standing motionless for long periods in a warm, airless place.

Symptoms and signs
- Sensations of heat, weakness, nausea and dizziness.
- Yawning.
- Pale, clammy skin.
- Slow, weak pulse.
- Collapse.

Treating fainting

1 Don't wait for the casualty to collapse, help him to lie down and immediately elevate the legs.

2 Loosen any tight clothing around the neck, chest and waist.

3 Turn the head to one side in case of vomiting.

4 Try to provide fresh air by opening a window or fanning the face, and keep onlookers back.

5 Consciousness is normally regained very quickly, but advise the casualty to remain lying down for at least 10 minutes.

6 If consciousness does not quickly return, check the breathing and pulse and be prepared to resuscitate if necessary (see pages 17-23).

7 If unconsciousness persists but breathing is present, place the casualty in the recovery position (see pages 25-26) and dial 999 for an ambulance.

Elevate the casualty's legs and turn the head to one side.

Feverish fit
(Febrile convulsion)

Fever is a feature of many childhood illnesses, and convulsions due to overheating are common in children below the age of 2 years. The situation is sometimes aggravated by a well-meaning parent wrapping up a feverish child too warmly. Although frightening for parents to witness, febrile convulsions are not life-threatening. However, they do require specific action.

Symptoms and signs

● There is often a short history of preceding illness such as a sore throat.
● Skin flushed and hot to touch, sometimes sweaty.
● Jerky movements of limbs with clenching of fists and arching of back.
● Eyes may be upturned or squinting.
● Breath-holding can occur with congestion of face and neck.

Over-breathing
(hyperventilation) attack

Although carbon dioxide is a waste-product that we exhale from our lungs, a certain quantity is necessary for health, and carbon dioxide levels in the bloodstream are carefully regulated by a special centre in the brain. In times of stress, the respiratory rate tends to increase and, if over-breathing continues for any length of time, unpleasant symptoms can develop as the carbon dioxide level in the blood falls. Eventually the casualty may collapse. Sufferers tend to be anxious individuals, and may be unaware that they have been over-breathing.

Treatment of feverish fit

1 Clear a space around the child and protect it from injury.
2 Try to provide fresh air, e.g. by opening a window.
3 Remove clothing and begin sponging the body with tepid water, but do not over-cool.

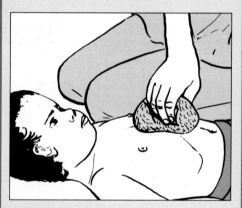

4 When the convulsions stop, place the child in the recovery position, reassure and cover lightly.
5 Telephone for a doctor in order to establish the cause of the high temperature.
6 Keep under observation in case a further fit occurs, and repeat steps 1 to 3 if necessary.

Symptoms and signs

● Feelings of panic, dizziness and tingling in the hands.
● Rapid, deep breathing.
● Trembling of hands.
● Spasm of muscles in the hands and feet.

Fractures, dislocations, sprains and strains

Bone is one of the hardest substances in the body, capable of withstanding great stresses. Yet bone is a living tissue, and all the bones of our skeleton possess a rich network of blood vessels and nerve fibres. This explains why, when a bone breaks, much pain, bleeding, swelling and bruising tend to occur.

Types of fracture

There is no difference between a fracture, a

Types of fracture

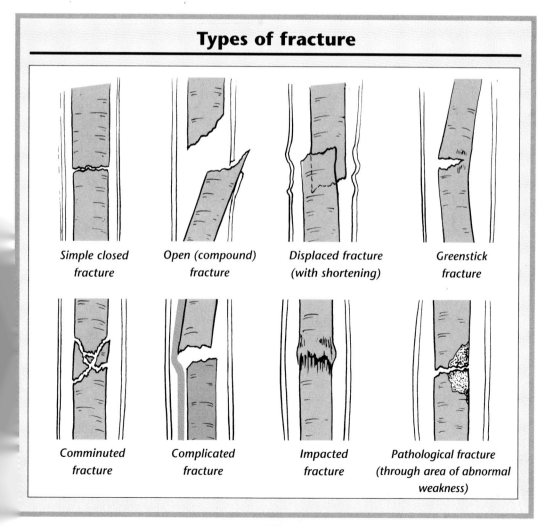

Simple closed fracture

Open (compound) fracture

Displaced fracture (with shortening)

Greenstick fracture

Comminuted fracture

Complicated fracture

Impacted fracture

Pathological fracture (through area of abnormal weakness)

break and a crack. There are several different types of fracture, break or crack, but the words themselves have the same meaning.

1 Closed fracture

In a closed fracture, the overlying skin remains intact.

2 Open fracture

An open (or compound) fracture is one in which the overlying skin is broken, a piece of bone often protruding through the wound. This allows germs to get to the fracture site, and subsequent infection can interfere with the healing process.

3 Displaced fracture

This is one where the ends of the broken bone are no longer in normal alignment. When displacement is severe, an operation may be required to fix the bone ends in a position where they can knit together.

4 Simple fracture

A simple fracture is one where there has been a single, clean break through the bone.

5 Greenstick fracture

As its name suggests, a greenstick fracture is one where the bone has not been completely divided. Greenstick fractures tend to occur in children, because their bones are more elastic than those of an adult.

6 Comminuted fracture

In a comminuted fracture, shattering at the fracture site results in a number of loose fragments.

7 Complicated fracture

This is one in which adjacent structures such as nerves, major blood vessels or organs have also been damaged.

8 Impacted fracture

At the time of the injury, if the broken bone

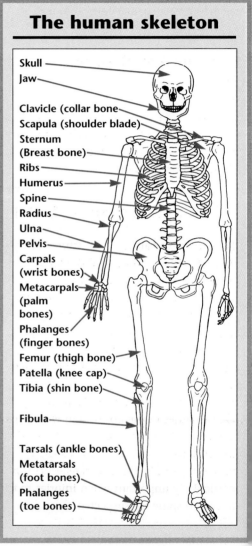

The human skeleton

Skull
Jaw
Clavicle (collar bone)
Scapula (shoulder blade)
Sternum (Breast bone)
Ribs
Humerus
Spine
Radius
Ulna
Pelvis
Carpals (wrist bones)
Metacarpals (palm bones)
Phalanges (finger bones)
Femur (thigh bone)
Patella (knee cap)
Tibia (shin bone)
Fibula
Tarsals (ankle bones)
Metatarsals (foot bones)
Phalanges (toe bones)

ends are driven into one another, the resulting fracture can be relatively stable. Pain and loss of function are often less marked when a fracture is impacted.

9 Pathological fracture

A pathological fracture is one which passes

through an abnormal area of bone, weakened by things like cysts, tumours or ageing (osteoporosis).

Symptoms and signs of a fracture

1 Snap
The casualty may report having heard, or felt, a snap at the time of the injury, but structures other than bone can sometimes do this.

2 Pain and tenderness
Pain is often severe and is aggravated by movement. Anything that reduces movement at the fracture site will ease pain.

3 Loss of function
Normal movement is limited by pain and instability.

4 Swelling and bruising
This is caused by bleeding from damaged blood vessels in the fractured bone. Swelling tends to occur quickly, whereas bruising may take some time to become obvious.

First Aid treatment of fractures – general principles

The First aid treatment of fractures to individual bones is beyond the scope of this book. Nevertheless, for the inexperienced First Aider, there are certain general principles of treatment that can be applied to all fractures.

They are as follows:

1 First ensure that it is safe to approach the casualty.

2 Whenever possible, try to treat casualties in the position in which they are found. Except for minor fractures of the upper limb, do not move the casualty unless he is in immediate danger - this is particularly important when injuries to the neck and spine are suspected.

3 If necessary, follow the A B C of resuscitation (see pages 17-23).

4 Treat any serious bleeding (see page 37).

5 Dial 999 for an ambulance.

6 Steady and support an injured limb by holding it above and below the fracture site. Alternatively, use cushions or folded clothing to support the injured part.

7 Do not attempt to straighten a fractured limb. You could make the injury worse, and you will certainly aggravate pain if the casualty is conscious.

8 Leave the application of lower limb splints to ambulance personnel. Careful manual support is always superior to a badly-applied splint.

9 Do not give the casualty anything to eat or drink, as he may require an general anaesthetic.

10 Whilst awaiting the ambulance, keep the casualty warm and monitor the breathing, pulse and level of consciousness.

11 If the casualty becomes unconscious, turn him into the recovery position (see pages 25-26), or resuscitate if necessary (see pages 17-23).

The A-Z of first aid

Sprains and strains

A sprain occurs when the fibres of a ligament are stretched and torn. Occasionally ligaments snap in two (ruptured ligament), but usually the tear is partial. With a severe sprain, damage to blood vessels around the ligament often results in rapid swelling of the joint, and it may be impossible to exclude a fracture without an X-ray. All severe sprains should therefore be referred to a doctor for examination. The ligament on the outer side of the ankle joint is frequently sprained, particularly in adolescent girls.

A strain refers to a tear in a muscle, or its tendon (the tough cord which joins muscle to bone), and the hamstring muscles at the back of the thigh are prone to strain injuries. Occasionally tendons may rupture completely, e.g. the Achilles tendon at the back of the ankle.

5 **Deformity**
The fracture of a bone in a limb can give it a twisted appearance (rotation), make it point in a unusual direction (angulation) or, when the bone ends override one another, produce shortening of the limb. Bones of the skull and face can be driven inwards, resulting in a depressed fracture.

6 **Grating (crepitus) of bone ends**
Crepitus should never be elicited deliberately, as movement at the fracture site will aggravate pain and bleeding, and could bring on shock. Careless movement could also damage vital structures causing a complicated fracture, or even convert a closed fracture into an open one.

Dislocations

At a joint, the adjacent bone ends are anchored together by strong bands called ligaments. These ligaments prevent the joint moving in abnormal directions, but violent twisting forces can tear the ligaments and allow the bone ends to become displaced.

The commonest joints to dislocate are those of the fingers, shoulder and ankle, but the First Aider should be aware that a fracture often accompanies a dislocation (known as a fracture-dislocation). Any dislocation of the vertebrae in the neck is particularly dangerous, since rough handling by a First Aider could cause damage to the spinal cord, resulting in death or permanent paralysis.

The First Aider should never attempt to put a dislocated joint back in place. Instead, the injury should be treated as though it were a fracture, and the casualty transferred to hospital.

Remember

Remembering the word RICE can help when treating minor sprains and strains:

Rest in the most comfortable position.
Ice pack applied for at least 30 minutes.
Compress with a crêpe bandage.
Elevate the affected part.

Head injuries and unconsciousness

The brain is a very delicate organ that is protected by the bony skull. Within the skull, it is suspended in a bath of fluid called cerebro-spinal fluid, which helps to absorb shock waves that would otherwise be transmitted directly to the brain. Most of the nerves of the body are connected to the brain by way of the spinal cord, which runs down the length of the spine within its own protective bony canal. The tissues of the brain and spinal cord are unable to repair themselves, so it is vital that they are protected from serious injury.

Fractures of the skull

A fracture of the skull signifies that violent forces have been applied to the head, but it is the damage to the underlying brain that is more important, since permanent brain damage or even death can follow a head injury where the skull has survived intact. Occasionally an area of the skull may be driven inwards (depressed fracture) compressing the brain beneath, and a

Signs of cerebral compression include:

- Headache, vomiting or yawning.
- Deteriorating level of consciousness, then unconsciousness.
- Pupils of different sizes. As compression increases, eventually both pupils become large and stop constricting to light.
- Weakness or paralysis of one side of the body.
- Isolated jerking of a limb or generalised convulsions.
- Breathing may be initially rapid, then slow and noisy.
- Slow, strong pulse.
- High temperature with flushed face.
- Respiratory arrest.

depressed fracture may initially be missed if bruising of the scalp has filled out the hollow in the skull surface. A fracture of the base of the skull can cause watery, blood-stained

Causes of unconsciousness

Cause	Examples
Reduction of blood supply to brain	Fainting, shock, stroke, cardiac arrest
Reduction of oxygen supply to brain	Suffocation, choking, carbon monoxide poisoning
Physical damage to brain	Concussion, compression, abnormal body temperature
Toxic damage to brain	Poisons, drugs
Other causes	Epilepsy, low blood sugar (hypoglycaemia)

fluid (cerebro-spinal fluid) to leak from a casualty's nose or ears.

Concussion and compression

Heavy blows to the head can disrupt normal brain function, resulting in a period of reduced consciousness or unconsciousness known as concussion. In addition, if there is bleeding or swelling within the rigid skull, the brain can be subjected to dangerous compression. Cerebral compression may take hours or even days to fully develop. This is why those who suffer head injuries often need a period of observation in hospital.

Unconsciousness

Unconsciousness is an abnormal state caused by a wide range of conditions that interrupt brain function. It differs from the normal sleeping state in that the subject cannot be fully roused. Unconsciousness is dangerous because the airway can become blocked by vomit, or obstructed by the tongue falling against the back of the throat.

Diagnosing unconsciousness

Gently shake the casualty's shoulders and shout, 'Are you all right?', but take care not to jerk the neck, in case there are spinal injuries. If the casualty does not respond to your voice, try the effect of pinching an earlobe, or rubbing a knuckle over the breastbone. If there is no response to voice or pain, then the casualty is unconscious.

First Aid treatment of unconsciousness

1 First ensure that it is safe to approach the casualty.

2 After confirming unconsciousness, open the Airway by tilting the head backwards and lifting the jaw (see page 12).

3 Look, listen and feel for signs of Breathing (see page 14).

4 Check the Circulation by feeling the carotid pulse, and resuscitate if necessary (see pages 17-23).

5 If the casualty is breathing and has a pulse, stop any serious bleeding (see page 37) and then stabilise any fractures.

6 Check for other injuries, e.g. look for bruises or wounds to the scalp that could suggest a head injury. Search for external clues like medical warning tags that might indicate the nature of the problem, and smell the breath for alcohol.

7 Providing the casualty is still breathing, turn him into the recovery position (see pages 25-26), but take great care if you suspect there may be a neck injury (see page 72).

8 Dial 999 for an ambulance if this has not already been done.

9 Continue to monitor the breathing and pulse, and be prepared to resuscitate if necessary.

10 Stay with the casualty until the ambulance arrives, and tell the crew of your findings.

Heart attack

The muscular wall of the heart (known as the myocardium) is fed by the coronary arteries, and serious problems arise if the blood flow in these vessels is interrupted.

Coronary artery disease

In certain individuals, the coronary arteries become progressively narrowed as fatty deposits build up on their inside walls. This process tends to restrict the blood supply to the heart muscle so that, when the heart is working hard, it can run short of oxygen. Those affected experience a cramp-like chest pain during exercise called angina, which is quickly relieved by rest. Angina sufferers are also be helped by a drug called glyceryl trinitrate (otherwise known as GTN or TNT) which come in aerosol form, or as tablets to be dissolved under the tongue.

A heart attack (or myocardial infarct) occurs when a blood clot forms inside a diseased coronary artery, an event known as a coronary thrombosis. As a result, the blood supply to a portion of heart muscle is suddenly cut off, and the muscle will die if the flow is not quickly restored. The victim may have a history of angina, but often the attack itself is the first sign of a heart problem. Sometimes it can be difficult to tell the difference between a mild heart attack and a bad attack of angina but, if the pain lasts for more than 15 minutes and is not relieved by rest or glyceryl trinitrate, a heart attack should always be suspected.

Around 60 per cent of victims survive a

Why do people develop coronary heart disease?

Narrowing of the coronary arteries is an inevitable consequence of ageing, but sometimes the process begins prematurely, and a number of precipitating causes – known as risk factors – have been identified. In addition to age, the risk factors for coronary artery disease include:

- Male gender.
- Family history of coronary artery disease.
- High blood cholesterol levels.
- Cigarette smoking.
- High blood pressure.
- Obesity.
- Diabetes.
- Lack of exercise.
- Diet high in saturated animal fat, low in fruit and fibre.
- Alcohol excess.
- Stress etc.

heart attack, scar tissue gradually replacing any dead or damaged muscle. However, research has shown that an aspirin tablet, given as soon as possible after the onset of symptoms, can significantly improve a victim's chances of survival. It is thought that aspirin works by inhibiting the clotting process within the affected coronary artery.

The A-Z of first aid

Cardiac arrest

During the early stages of a heart attack, the dying portion of heart muscle becomes very irritable, and this irritability can suddenly spread to involve the rest of the heart, causing it to go into spasm and stop beating. This condition is called ventricular fibrillation, and it often occurs within minutes of the onset of the attack. Ventricular fibrillation can be easily reversed with the aid of a special machine called a defibrillator, carried on most emergency ambulances. If cardio-pulmonary resuscitation (CPR) has been started immediately, the chances of successful defibrillation are high.

Symptoms and signs of a heart attack

During a heart attack, a number of symptoms and signs may occur, including:
1 Severe pain in the chest in virtually all cases. The pain of a heart attack usually comes on gradually over a period of minutes, building into a severe, crushing pain in the centre of the chest. It may radiate up to the throat and jaw, through to the back, or out to the shoulders and down the inside of the arms. The pain is similar to that of angina, but tends to be much more severe, and is not relieved by rest or glyceryl trinitrate.
2 Pallor or greyness of the skin which also feels cold and clammy.
3 Weakness and dizziness.
4 Breathlessness.
5 Nausea and vomiting.
6 Sudden collapse (low blood pressure or cardiac arrest).

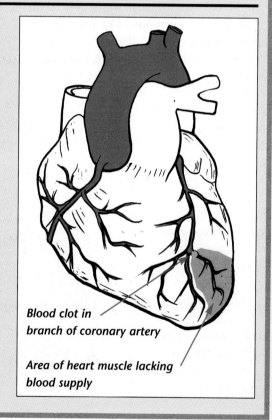

Blood clot in branch of coronary artery

Area of heart muscle lacking blood supply

EMERGENCY ACTION

Heart attack

THE PULSE is likely to be weak and rapid (over 100 beats/minute), and is often irregular; but it may also be slow (under 50 beats/minute), and is sometimes normal. If the casualty loses consciousness and the carotid pulse disappears, cardiac arrest has occurred, and full CPR must be started immediately (see pages 21-23).

1 Help the casualty into a half-sitting position and place pillows or folded clothing behind his head and shoulders, and under his knees. Loosen any tight clothing.

2 Shout for help, or go yourself to dial 999 for an ambulance. Make it clear that you think the casualty is having a heart attack.

3 If the casualty is conscious, give him an aspirin tablet to chew, followed by a sip of water.

4 Whilst waiting for the ambulance, monitor the breathing and pulse, and be prepared to resuscitate if necessary.

Recommended item

- Aspirin (300mg)

IMPORTANT

- Do not allow the casualty to move as this could upset the heart rhythm.
- If the heart stops, the casualty will lose consciousness within seconds. He may take gasping breaths for a short time, but CPR should be started immediately.
- Do not give aspirin if there is a history of serious allergy to this drug.

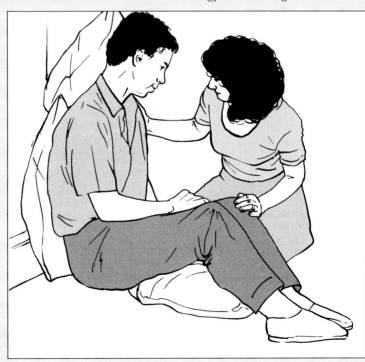

Nosebleeds

Nosebleeds are very common and are rarely serious.

They occur:

- After a direct blow to the nose.
- During infections like colds and 'flu.
- As a result of sneezing, nose-picking or heavy blowing of the nose.
- Spontaneously.

Recurrent, spontaneous nosebleeds usually indicate a weak, prominent blood vessel inside a nostril, and sufferers can sometimes benefit from cautery, where the offending vessel is shrivelled by means of the painless application of an electrical current, or caustic chemical. In young children, a persistent, blood-stained, smelly discharge from one nostril often signals the presence of a foreign body, such as a plastic bead, in the nose. After a bad head injury, a blood-stained, watery discharge from the nose can be a sign of a skull fracture.

Treatment of a nosebleed

1 Sit the casualty down with his head bent forward over a bowl or wash-basin. Reassure him and loosen any tight clothing around the neck.

2 Advise the casualty to breath through his mouth, whilst firmly pinching the soft part of the nose, just below the bone, between thumb and index finger. Tell him to avoid swallowing any blood that trickles down the back of the throat, as this can cause nausea and vomiting. Give him a tissue to mop up any blood that dribbles from the mouth.

3 Pressure should be applied for a full 10 minutes. If bleeding persists, apply pressure for a further 10 minutes. If control is not achieved within 30 minutes, maintain pressure and consult a doctor.

4 When bleeding stops, carefully clean around the nose and mouth using a swab soaked in lukewarm water, and advise the casualty to rest quietly and avoid blowing the nose for the next 4 hours.

5 If the bleeding resulted from an direct blow, and the nose appears to be crooked, consult a doctor immediately as there may be a nasal fracture which needs to be straightened.

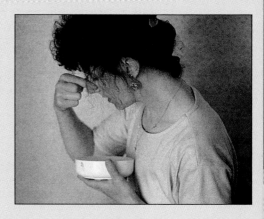

Poisoning

A poison can be defined as any substance that exerts a harmful effect on the body. The damage done may be either temporary or permanent, and the toxicity usually depends on the quantity taken. Poisoning may be accidental or deliberate. When a large quantity of a medicine is deliberately taken in a suicide attempt, the casualty is said to have taken an 'overdose'.

Prevention of poisoning
● Always place household poisons out of the reach of children.
● Never store chemicals in bottles which originally held soft drinks.
● Keep all medicines in their original containers in a locked cabinet.
● Never share prescribed medicines with another person.

How poisons enter the body

Route	Examples
By mouth (oral route)	Overdose of paracetamol/ bleach taken by child
By inhalation	Fumes containing carbon monoxide
By absorption through skin	Sprays containing pesticides and insecticides
By injection beneath skin	Illicit drugs / bee stings and snake bites

● Be aware that alcohol can potentiate the harmful effects of many medicines.

Poisoning

Poison or drug	Harmful effects	Comments
Alcohol	'Drunkenness', nausea, vomiting, coma, hypothermia, respiratory arrest.	Inhalation of vomit a serious risk. If unconscious, place casualty in recovery position, but DO NOT ABANDON. Beware of unrecognised head injury.
Amphetamines including amphetamine derivatives like 'Ecstasy'.	Wakefulness, hyperactivity, belligerence, agitation, sweating, tremor of hands, rapid pulse, large pupils, overheating, convulsions, cardiac arrest (rare).	Fashionable drugs at 'rave' parties. Sometimes injected. Effects may last several hours.

Continued on page 70

The A-Z of first aid

Poisoning

Continued from page 69

Poison or drug	Harmful effects	Comments
Antidepressants	Effects vary according to type of drug taken. Coma, convulsions, respiratory and cardiac arrest all possible.	Try to identify drug in question and inform ambulance personnel or doctor. Worse when mixed with alcohol.
Aspirin	Ringing in ears (tinnitus), headache, nausea, sweating, rapid breathing, overheating, coma, convulsions.	Many over-the-counter preparations contain aspirin. Vomit may contain blood.
Carbon monoxide (CO)	Cherry-pink skin, coma, respiratory arrest.	Immediately evacuate casualty into fresh air. CO blocks uptake of oxygen in blood, starving brain of oxygen.
Cocaine	Overdose effects similar to amphetamines but much shorter-acting (around $1/2$ hour).	Sniffed, smoked or injected. 'Crack' cocaine is highly addictive.
Corrosive agents **Acids:** battery acid, metal polishes, rust removers, toilet bowl cleaners. **Alkalis:** ammonia, bleach, dishwasher detergents, drain cleaners, oven cleaners, washing soda.	Burns to skin, mouth, throat, gullet (oesophagus) and stomach.	Give sips of milk or water if conscious. Wash agent from skin thoroughly. DO NOT INDUCE VOMITING. Transport in sitting position.
Hallucinogens e.g. LSD and 'magic mushrooms'.	Agitation, flushed skin, large pupils, nausea, vomiting, hallucinations, delirium, paranoia, coma.	Protect casualty from accidental self-injury. First Aider may need to reassure someone having a bad 'trip'.
Hydrocarbons e.g. diesel oil, paraffin, lighter fluid, paint thinners, petrol.	Abdominal pain, cough, severe breathing problems, convulsions, coma, respiratory arrest.	DO NOT INDUCE VOMITING. Transport in sitting position.
Iron preparations	Abdominal pain, nausea, vomiting, diarrhoea, intestinal bleeding.	Treat for shock if necessary.
Narcotics e.g. heroin, opium, morphine.	Small or pinpoint pupils, drowsiness, confusion, coma, respiratory arrest.	Usually smoked or taken by injection. Look for fresh injection marks (usually around elbows, wrists or hands).

Poisoning

Poison or drug	Harmful effects	Comments
Paracetamol	Little effect initially, then possible liver failure days later, leading to coma and death.	Treatment within 12 hours can prevent liver damage.
Plant poisons e.g. deadly nightshade, foxglove, fungi (various), laburnum, yew.	Effects vary according to plant species, but include abdominal pain, nausea, vomiting and convulsions.	Take or send a specimen of plant to hospital with casualty.
Sleeping tablets and tranquillisers	Drowsiness, confusion, coma, respiratory arrest.	Worse when mixed with alcohol.
Solvents etc. (inhaled) e.g. aerosols, glue, butane gas.	Cough, dizziness, drowsiness, headache, nausea, vomiting, choking, cardiac arrest (rare).	A glue-sniffer will sometimes have spots around his mouth or nose. Never chase solvent misusers around or over-excite them, as it can precipitate cardiac arrest.

General aspects of management

● Try to find out WHAT was taken, WHEN it was taken, and HOW MUCH was taken.
● Never attempt to induce vomiting, except rarely when directed to do so by a doctor. In particular never induce vomiting in someone who has swallowed an acid, alkali or hydrocarbon or in someone who is semi-conscious or unconscious, and never give salt water to induce vomiting – it is a poison in its own right.
● Where appropriate, send empty bottles, tablets, plant specimens and vomit with the casualty to hospital.
● Be prepared to follow the ABC of resuscitation, if necessary (see pages 17-23).

Spinal injuries

The spine, or backbone, is a column of bones called vertebrae, which are held together by strong ligaments. In total there are 33 vertebrae grouped into five distinct regions.

Within the spine, the delicate spinal cord occupies its own bony canal where it is protected from damage. The spinal cord is really a huge bundle of nerve fibres, some carrying instructions from the brain to make muscles move (motor fibres), and others carrying messages back to the brain concerning sensations such as heat and pain (sensory fibres).

If the spinal cord is severed, this results

The A-Z of first aid

in permanent paralysis and total loss of all sensation below the level of the injury. When such an injury occurs high in the neck, the outcome is usually fatal since all the breathing muscles are immediately paralysed. It is vitally important therefore, that all casualties with spinal injuries are handled with extreme caution. A casualty

The spinal recovery position

When neck injuries are suspected an unconscious casualty should only be turned into the recovery position if there are signs that vomiting is about to occur. Ideally, two or more people should turn the casualty, and one person should be solely responsible for keeping the head and neck in line with the body. The spinal recovery position is identical to the standard recovery position (see pages 25-26), except that the head and neck are supported in an anatomical position until the ambulance arrives.

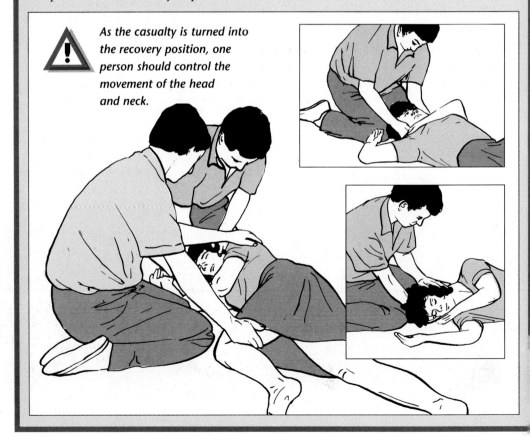

As the casualty is turned into the recovery position, one person should control the movement of the head and neck.

who has sustained neck injuries should not be moved unless there is immediate danger to life, e.g. from fire. Even then, every effort should be made to support the neck.

Symptoms of spinal injury

A conscious casualty with spinal injuries may complain of:

- Pain or stiffness in the spine at the level of the injury.
- Tingling, burning, shooting pains or numbness below the level of the injury.
- Weakness of, or an inability to move, the limbs.

Management of the unconscious casualty

When a casualty is unconscious, it is often impossible to know whether or not spinal injuries have been sustained, as the victim is unable report numbness and weakness. It is therefore safer to assume that all casualties who are unconscious as a result of head injuries, have also sustained spinal damage. In particular, beware of incidents where the casualty has fallen head-first from a height, e.g. gymnasts, trampolinists and those who accidentally dive into shallow water.

When treating casualties with suspected spinal injuries, the priorities remain:

A A clear Airway.
B Adequate Breathing.
C An effective Circulation.

But be careful to use only the minimum amount of movement necessary when tilting the head backwards to open the airway.

Management of conscious casualty

1 Reassure the casualty and tell him not to move.

2 Steady and support the head, keeping the head and neck in a straight line with the body. On no account should you allow the neck to twist or bend.

3 Send a bystander to dial 999 for an ambulance. If you are on your own, first place convenient items like folded clothing on either side of the casualty to support the head, neck and shoulders.

4 Continue to steady and support the head until the ambulance arrives. Home made splints for the neck are not effective and it is far better simply to maintain manual control of the head and neck preventing movement. There is no point in risking doing damage applying an ineffective splint which will have to be removed by ambulance personnel on their arrival.

The A-Z of first aid

Extremes of temperature

The human body functions best at temperatures between 36 and 37.5°C (97-99°F), and the core temperature is kept within this range by a heat-regulation centre in the brain. Body heat is generated by the conversion of food into thermal energy, supplemented by heat produced during muscular activity.

The body's response to cold

In cold weather, body heat is preserved by a reflex mechanism which shuts down blood vessels in the skin and, although the skin itself goes pale and cold, the loss of precious core heat to the surroundings is cut to a minimum. Involuntary muscular activity in the form of shivering then begins to generate extra heat. Furry animals fluff out their coats to improve insulation, and humans also have small muscles attached to hairs in the skin, which make them stand up in 'goose pimples' in response to cold. We supplement these natural mechanisms by dressing warmly, taking hot food and drink, seeking shelter in warm surroundings and flexing our muscles. A continuing loss of body heat eventually results in a condition called hypothermia, to which both babies and the elderly are particularly susceptible.

Hypothermia

A casualty is considered to be suffering from hypothermia when the core temperature drops below 35°C (95°F). As the body temperature falls towards 35°C, the victim is still aware of being extremely cold but, once below this level, the overwhelming feeling is one of apathy. As the body temperature continues to fall, victims become increasingly confused and, at temperatures below 32°C (90°F), some people may even attempt to undress because of a sensation of heat. A core temperature below 30°C (85°F) indicates severe hypothermia; the muscles become rigid and the casualty slips towards unconsciousness. At 27°C (81°F), there may be few signs of life, with no discernible pulse and shallow respirations down to as few as 2 or 3 a minute. A further reduction in temperature eventually brings about ventricular fibrillation, and the heart stops beating.

The body's response to heat

To prevent the body overheating in hot weather, blood vessels in the skin are made to open up. The skin becomes flushed and feels warm to the touch, and excess heat is radiated to the surroundings. At the same time, glands in the skin secrete sweat, which cools the skin surface as it evaporates. Panting also helps to get rid of warm breath from the lungs, replacing it with cooler, inspired air. We then assist these reflex changes by removing clothing, drinking cool liquids, seeking shade and avoiding exertion. Heavy sweating can lead to heat exhaustion but, if sweating ceases, there is a risk of heat-stroke.

Heat exhaustion

Heat exhaustion occurs when the body loses

excessive quantities of water and salt as a result of heavy sweating. After suddenly collapsing, the casualty often remains reasonably alert, and may complain of weakness, muscle cramps, headache, dizziness and nausea.

Signs of heat exhaustion
- Complexion pale or grey.
- Skin cool and moist.
- Pulse weak and rapid.
- Signs of shock may be present if dehydration is severe (see page 36).

Heat-stroke
Heat-stroke occurs when the body suddenly loses its ability to sweat, allowing a rapid rise in body temperature. Classic heat-stroke occurs during a heat wave and tends to affect the elderly, when chronic illness and dehydration may play a part. In Britain, however, heat-stroke usually follows

Treatment of heat exhaustion

1 Lie the casualty down in a cool place and elevate the legs.
2 Give repeated sips of a weak solution of salt water (1 level 5 ml teaspoonful of salt per litre), until the casualty's condition improves.
3 Call a doctor for further advice.

sustained, vigorous exercise in hot, humid weather. Victims of exertional heat-stroke often collapse suddenly in a state of mental confusion, and may lapse into coma or suffer convulsions. Temperatures over 41°C (105°F) are not tolerated for long, and mortality rates are high unless rapid cooling can be effected. The casualty will appear flushed and have a rapid, strong pulse and a hot, dry skin.

Features of heat exhaustion and heat-stroke

	Heat exhaustion	Exertional heat-stroke
History of exertion	Sometimes	Yes
Collapse	Often Sudden	Sudden
Mental state	Usually alert	Confused/delirious
Convulsions	Rare	Common
Skin temperature	Normal or cool	Hot
Skin colour	Pale or grey	Flushed
Skin moisture	Moist	Dry
Pulse	Rapid and weak	Rapid and strong

The A-Z of first aid

Treatment of hypothermia

1 Prevent further heat loss by bringing the casualty indoors, or by finding shelter from the elements. Remove any wet garments and replace with warm, dry clothing.

2 If indoors, and providing the casualty can move unaided, immerse in a hot bath at 40C (104F). If outdoors, protect the casualty from the wind, insulate from cold ground, and try to keep him dry.

3 Providing the casualty is conscious, give hot sweet drinks, if available. Under no circumstances should alcohol be given, as it has the effect of aggravating hypothermia.

4 If the casualty's condition deteriorates, dial 999 for an ambulance. Be prepared to resuscitate if necessary (see pages 17-23), but check the carotid pulse for at least 30 seconds before diagnosing cardiac arrest.

IMPORTANT

● In severe hypothermia, where the casualty has blue or ice-cold skin, stiff or rigid muscles and is behaving irrationally or is unconscious, handle very gently and NEVER apply heat, as cardiac arrest may result.

● Death cannot be reliably diagnosed in hypothermia until after re-warming has been accomplished.

Treatment of heat-stroke

1 Try to find a cool, breezy place to lie the casualty down, and remove all outer garments.

2 Wrap the casualty in a cold, wet sheet, and keep the sheet saturated by sprinkling or pouring cold water over it. Fan the sheet as much as possible.

3 Continue cooling until the skin feels cool, or until the body temperature falls to 38C (100.4F).

4 Beware of a second rise in body temperature, and be prepared to repeat steps 1 to 3 if necessary. Advise the casualty to lie quietly in a cool place until fully recovered.

Recommended items
● Watering can.
● Cold water.
● Thin, cotton sheet.

IMPORTANT

● If the casualty becomes unconscious, check breathing and pulse, and be prepared to resuscitate if necessary (see pages 17-23).

● An unconscious casualty who is breathing should be placed in the recovery position (see pages 25-26).

Recommended items for a First Aid kit

First Aid kits are widely available, or individual items can be purchased separately and stored in any suitable container with an air-tight lid (e.g. an ice-cream carton or sandwich box).

Item	Size etc.	Comments
Adhesive dressings	Assorted	Waterproof plasters best for hand wounds
Adhesive tape	1 roll (2.5cm wide)	Hypo-allergenic paper tape recommended e.g. 'Micropore'
Conforming bandages (e.g. 'Kling')	1 (5cm) 1 (7.5cm)	Useful for light bandaging, where firm pressure not required
Cotton wool balls	1 packet	For cleaning wounds, etc.
Cotton wool roll	1 roll	For padding. Do not apply directly to wounds
Crêpe bandages	1 (5cm) 1 (7.5cm)	For pressure bandaging to control bleeding and swelling
Eye bandage (sterile)	1	
Field dressing (sterile)	1 large size	For covering large wounds
First Aid book		
Gauze swabs (sterile)	2 packs of 10 (10cm²)	For applying pressure over bleeding wounds, cleaning wounds etc.
Non-stick dressings (sterile) (e.g. 'Melolin')	3 (5cm²) 3 (10cm²)	Less likely to stick to wound than plain gauze. Apply shiny surface to wound
Paraffin gauze dressings (e.g. 'Jelonet')	1 tin of 10 pieces (10cm²)	For burns and grazes. Prevents dressing sticking to wound
Triangular bandages	2	For slings. Can be folded into bandage
Tubular gauze finger dressings		Available as ready-to-apply units, or in roll for use with applicator
Antiseptic solution (e.g. 'Savlon')	1 bottle (plastic)	For cleaning wounds and instruments
Dish (small)	1	Small foil cake case makes excellent disposable container for antiseptic solution
Disposable plastic gloves	2 pairs	To minimize cross-infection
Pencil and writing pad	1	Handy in an emergency
Safety pins	Various sizes	
Scissors	1 pr. pointed, 1 pr. blunt-ended	Blunt-ended scissors prevent injury when removing dressings etc.
Thermometer (clinical)		Mercury bulb, electronic or disposable types available.
Tweezers	Flat-ended	(without serrations) For removing splinters, etc.

The A-Z of first aid

Medicines for the home

Consult your local pharmacist for further advice on home remedies, and remember to keep all medicines in a locked cabinet out of the reach of children.

Problem	Medicine	Comments
Acid indigestion	Antacid tablets or liquid	Consult your doctor if symptoms persist
Blocked nose	Decongestant spray Antihistamines may also help	Do not use decongestant sprays for extended periods
Cold sores	5% acyclovir cream	Apply as soon as symptoms start
Constipation	Lactulose solution Senna tablets (adults) Glycerine suppositories (rectal use)	Consult doctor if problem persists
Cough	Cough linctus	Hot honey and lemon drink probably just as effective
Diarrhoea	Loperamide capsules or syrup Kaolin mixture Rehydration sachets (children)	Beware of dehydration in young children, especially when child is also vomiting
Fever	Paracetamol tablets or paediatric syrup Soluble aspirin tablets (adults)	Avoid aspirin in children below the age of 12 years
Heart attack	Aspirin tablet (300mg)	See page 67
Hay fever	Antihistamine tablets or syrup	Some preparations can cause drowsiness. Avoid alcohol
Insect bites/stings	1% Hydrocortisone cream	Avoid eyes
Migraine	See under 'Pain'	'Femigraine' or 'Migraleve' may also help
Pain	Paracetamol tablets or paediatric syrup Soluble aspirin tablets (adults) Ibuprofen tablets or syrup	Avoid aspirin in children below the age of 12 years. Ibuprofen can help when inflammation is causing pain
Rashes (itchy)	Calamine lotion Antihistamine tablets or syrup	For small areas try 1% hydrocortisone cream, but consult doctor if rash spreads
Sore throat	Throat lozenges. Antiseptic gargles	Antibiotics are sometimes necessary
Spots & infected wounds	Antiseptic cream	Antibiotics are sometimes necessary
Sprains & muscular aches	Ibuprofen tablets, gel or cream	Stop if tablets cause indigestion
Sunburn	Calamine lotion	Cool shower can also help

Useful information

BASICS
British Association for Immediate Care
7 Black Horse Lane
Ipswich
Suffolk IP1 2EF
Tel: 0473 218407

British Diabetic Association
10 Queen Anne Street
London W1M 0BD
Tel: 071 323 1531

British Heart Foundation
14 Fitzhardinge Street
London W1H 4DH
Tel: 071 935 0185

British Red Cross Society
28 Worple Road
Wimbledon
London SW19 4EE
Tel: 081 944 8909

Headway National Head Injuries Association Ltd
200 Mansfield Road
Nottingham NG1 3HX
Tel: 0602 622382

Medic Alert Foundation
12 Bridge Wharf
156 Caledonian Road
London N1 9UU
Tel: 071 833 3034

National Society for Epilepsy
Chalfont Centre for Epilepsy
Chalfont St Peter
Gerrards Cross
Bucks SL9 0RJ
Tel: 0240 73991

Release (the National Drugs and Legal Helpline)
169 Commercial Street
London
Tel: 071 377 5905
24-hour emergency line: 071 603 8654

Spinal Injuries Association
76 St James's Lane
London N10 3DF
Tel: 081 444 2121

St John Ambulance Brigade
1 Grosvenor Crescent
London SW1X 7EF
Tel: 071 235 5231

Index